Healing with Source

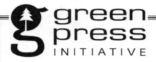

green press
I N I T I A T I V E

Findhorn Press is committed to preserving ancient forests and natural resources. We elected to print this title on 30% post consumer recycled paper, processed chlorine free. As a result, for this printing, we have saved:

5 Trees (40' tall and 6-8" diameter)
2 Million BTUs of Total Energy
518 Pounds of Greenhouse Gases
2,497 Gallons of Wastewater
152 Pounds of Solid Waste

Findhorn Press made this paper choice because our printer, Thomson-Shore, Inc., is a member of Green Press Initiative, a nonprofit program dedicated to supporting authors, publishers, and suppliers in their efforts to reduce their use of fiber obtained from endangered forests.

For more information, visit www.greenpressinitiative.org

Environmental impact estimates were made using the Environmental Defense Paper Calculator. For more information visit: www.papercalculator.org.

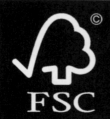

Mixed Sources
Product group from well-managed forests and other controlled sources
www.fsc.org   Cert no. SW-COC-002673
© 1996 Forest Stewardship Council

Healing with Source

A Spiritual Guide
to Mind-Body Medicine

Dave Markowitz

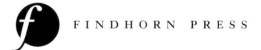

FINDHORN PRESS

The right of Dave Markowitz to be
identified as the author of this work has been asserted by him
in accordance with the Copyright, Designs and Patents Act 1998.

Published in 2010 by Findhorn Press, Scotland

ISBN 978-1-84409-511-7

A CIP record for this title is available from the British Library.

Edited by Nicky Leach
Cover design by Richard Crookes
Interior design by Damian Keenan
Printed and bound in the USA

Healing with Source Symbol ©2010 Janet Cristenfeld,
www.souligraphy.com
Author Photo © 2010 Christina Weber,
www.christinaweber.com

1 2 3 4 5 6 7 8 9 17 16 15 14 13 12 11 10

Published by

Findhorn Press

117-121 High Street,

Forres IV36 1AB,

Scotland, UK

t +44 (0)1309 690582

f +44 (0)131 777 2711

e info@findhornpress.com

www.findhornpress.com

Contents

Acknowledgments

In chronological order: Source, Mom, Dad, Sid, Carol, Mazzas, Levins, Richmans, Salty, Marc, Felix, Barry, Simon, the Lees, Paul, Dr. Michael Ryce, Dr. Bill, Faceboy, Dr. Yuen, Merry Miller, Mark Becker, Arthur Reel, Dr. Meg, Devra Ann Jacobs, Karin Knoblich, Andrea, Budly, Laurelle, Erin, Andrew, Shira Plotzker, Amy, everyone at BMSE, Yehuda Ashkenazi, Hillel Black, Nicky Leach, Thierry Bogliolo, and a special thank you to Joan D'Arcy.

Also to Goddesses Joanne D., Dara K., Tonya M., Maria S., Francesca C., Reina T., Rebecca C., and Tanis K.—Thank you.

Disclaimer

This manuscript is an accumulation of wisdom from both traditional and nontraditional sources. It is not intended to diagnose, cure, prevent, or treat your symptoms, disease, illness, or the like, or to diagnose or replace your medical treatment in any way, shape, or form, but merely to the introduce the reader to nontraditional ways of looking at things. Dave Markowitz, the editors, literary agent, book distributors/publishers/sellers, web-designer/hosting company, and others associated with Dave's work, make no medical claims whatsoever and assume no liability of any kind for the (mis)interpretation or (mis)implementation of this text, either written or implied. Simply use what resonates with you and discard the rest. Remember, it's always best to see your doctor.

IN LOVING MEMORY,
THIS BOOK IS DEDICATED TO
STEVEN LEVIN & MATILDA MAZZA.

Preface

How many of you have been pursuing the seemingly elusive goal of health? Like a dog chasing his own tail, it's just a tad out of reach. How many books, workshops, practitioners, and medications have you sought? How much money and time have you spent—and you're still not healthy!? Clearly, up until now, something has been amiss. You're about to learn what that "something" is and what you can do about it!

It is time to stop following outdated and insular ideas about health and healing. It is time to wake up to a new paradigm. I'm going to present you with a detailed map of understanding, preventing, and healing pain and illness. Each concept will build upon the previous idea, so it's important not to jump ahead. This journey may not prove easy, but the message is simple: stop doing what doesn't work and start doing what does. Are you ready for your A-HA moment?

As a medical intuitive with more than a decade of experience using the mind-body paradigm, I have seen people's lives make radical shifts following rules that have been given to me in meditations. Years of pain have vanished in just a few sessions, sometimes in just a few minutes. While you certainly have heard of mind-body medicine, it's never been presented quite like this before.

Health, like life, is a process. It is not a destination to set goals toward, but more a given end result from living consciously, being aware of how things work, what is missing, and where and how to fill in those blanks. That is what *Healing with Source: A Spiritual Guide to Mind-Body Medicine* will help you do.

Not *despite* but rather *in addition to* any evidence that says otherwise, my experience has shown that pain and illness come from within. Once we can accept that level of responsibility, a whole new world of living well and healing will open itself up to you. You'll want to try everything written here because, intrinsically, you will come to believe what you read is true. Any doubts that may arise will be addressed. Breathe, relax, and be open.

When prompted, gently tear or cut out the symbol on page 173 to use as a tool to assist you in the healing process; instructions are in Chapter 23. Notes symbolized by ✪ are interspersed as a reminder to claim your birthright of joy, and posted at *www.davemarkowitz.com/integrate* is an interlude of music that is subliminally encoded with each chapter's highlights, read by the author, to further integrate the information.

You are the key to healing yourself. And you are also the lock that must be opened. All of it is encompassed within you.

Enjoy!

Introduction

"Many are called but few are chosen" should be,
"All are called but few choose to listen."
—*A COURSE IN MIRACLES*

I am a work-in-progress, as are all of you. We are all on a journey. The Healing with Source work I do has been revealed to me slowly over a number of years, and I am still learning what it means to me and its relationship to the world. My hope is that you will join me on this path of discovery and find the Inner Healer that exists in all of you, then share this with the world.

I first became aware of the energy field while watching an alternative healthcare practitioner work with muscle testing. Muscle testing works by "asking" the body certain questions through specific movements. A muscle's relative strength or weakness determines what strengthens or weakens that person's energy field.

For example, let's say John has a neck pain. John holds his arm out to his side, and while the practitioner says out loud "anger at your mother" he pushes down on John's arm. John consciously offers moderate resistance. If the muscle stays strong, it indicates that anger at his mother is not the cause of the neck pain—in other words, that thought doesn't weaken his energy field. If the practitioner then says "anger at your father" and the muscle becomes weak—meaning the arm can be easily pushed down—then that indicates that anger at his father makes his energy field weaken. You then have the underlying cause of the neck pain identified. In order to really heal, you'll have to work through the repressed anger at Dad, even if it's decades old!

I watched the practitioner several times before I even believed what was happening. My big A-HA moment came when I took one of his classes, though. This time, instead of making a statement to determine strength or weakness, he asked a "yes or no" question, then began the muscle test. It became clear in that instant that he was communicating with a consciousness external of himself. I was determined to figure who or what this was!

I "borrowed" a friend's arm and began "asking" questions of the body, determined that I would become clear on what was happening at last! As I did the muscle testing, I intuitively felt a grandmother-type energy, and ascertained from the muscle test that it was, indeed, my grandmother's presence with me. Wow! She relayed a few things to me, including the information that it was not possible for me to understand her state of existence in that moment. Even without those details, there was a sense of peace from her, and maybe that was all I needed.

My friend's arm grew weary of this, so I asked other friends to lend me an ear, or arm, as it were. And then after annoying everyone else I was forced to learn self-testing. Eventually I was able to receive yes or no answers to very direct questions. One of my goals was to find out who or what else could be responding! I stayed awake nights communicating about seemingly everything (which became the basis for this book) but could never determine what was responding through yes or no questions alone. So I named it Peri. That name seemed innocuous and androgynous and somehow quite fitting.

I didn't tell too many people about this, of course. I barely believed it myself and feared the reactions of other people, just as I think most of us would in this situation. A few years later, I looked up "peri" in the dictionary. As a prefix it meant *around, about, all-encompassing,* and *enclosing,* as in the word "pericardium," meaning the membranous sac enclosing the heart. Quite fitting, wouldn't you say? I later learned that the proper noun Peri means a beautiful, benevolent supernatural being or fairy in Persian mythology! Pretty sweet, huh?

As time went on I started becoming more comfortable with this connection, though still didn't stand up and scream about it. And one day I got a feeling I was talking to something quite larger than I'd been led to believe: the Real Deal; the Big Cheese; El Jefe Grande! So I closed my eyes in fear of hearing an answer of yes and asked, "Are you God?" and I very calmly received a yes answer.

"Why me?" I wondered. (I wondered this a lot.)

> *Why is it when we talk to God, we are praying,*
> *but when God talks to us, we are called schizophrenic?*
> —*LILY TOMLIN, COMEDIENNE*

I felt I lacked the things I used to think were necessary to have a connection like this with God. I certainly didn't have a long white beard, a wardrobe of robes and sandals, or even any semblance of peace of mind. (When I grew facial hair it could barely be seen, and I never felt a need for a bathrobe, sandals, or even flip-flops, and could barely feign an air of contentment with myself, others, or life in general.) I also had lacked experiences with what we're told to believe are the keys to happiness, such as abundant finances or quality relationships, both romantic and otherwise.

In fact, I've run the gamut with things we're supposed to believe in. Being raised Jewish and taught to worship God in that particular way always left me with more questions than the incomplete and dubious answers that have been repeated for centuries by well-meaning scholars and lay people. Eventually, I saw how some organized religions indirectly invite seekers of deeper meaning toward agnosticism. Who hasn't wondered how a God could exist and let "his" children suffer so much? Though still hopeful of finding truth, my doubts soon outweighed all else.

The alternative healthcare practitioner who turned me on to energy healing work did not believe in God. Having witnessed his groundbreaking work, I trusted this man more than I did myself, so I, too, became an atheist. Though saddened by this version of reality, I allowed it to take over for a while, concluding that we're all a bunch of deranged lunatics wandering the planet with no rhyme or reason in search of a punchline to bring it all home. And that none could be found.

We are usually convinced more easily by reasons we have found ourselves
than by those which have occurred to others.
—*BLAISE PASCAL, MATHEMATICIAN AND PHILOSOPHER (1623–1662)*

Many years later, I more clearly understood what the practitioner meant when he said he didn't believe in "God." God as described by the old texts was a human projection based on a five-sensory reality that used logic and tangibility as co-factors in the equations used to understand, label, and explain reality. This man was trying to explain to us that God, for him, was an entity that is much more magnificent and benevolent. And now, through a long, arduous path of belief, questioning, doubt, denial, and a resurgence of faith via experience, I too have come to know this (re)source.

It is no accident that my spiritual path perfectly mirrors my path toward practicing mind-body medicine. I am no different from any of you. What started out for me as a solely tangible approach to health and illness—feeling unwell, going to the doctor, getting a prescription, feeling better—became a much more inclusive and holistic view when the limitations of conventional medicine were made clear. We're not a healthy people.

Moreover, if you believe that the energy that many people call by the name "God" is mean, you will have the view that we have no right in thinking we ever can be healthy—or even happy. But if you believe that God is more benevolent than what we've been taught, it follows that health and happiness are our birthrights!

I had to fight my doubts just to get through a series of classes, study, readings, conversations, meditations, and the like to get to this point. I had trouble believing in Shiatsu,

Therapeutic Touch, Muscle Testing, Touch for Health, Deep Emotional Release Work, Chakra Balancing, Channeling, Auras, Energy/Faith Healing, Crystal Therapy, prayer, and many other healing modalities. Now, these are as normal to me as taking an aspirin is for most of the population.

This is why I can empathize with you, dear reader, client, and workshop attendee who are having doubts about existential reality and even mind-body medicine. I've been there, done that. I understand many of your questions because I've asked them myself. And now that I'm intuitive, I can answer them before you ask! (That was a joke, by the way.)

This higher power (re)connection was terribly exciting and troublesome, scary and intriguing, all at once. After going through it, I asked myself, What would I now be directed to do? What had I done in my past lives to deserve this? Why did it take more than 30 years to happen? How can I tell anyone about it? Is everything I ever wanted now not only a possibility but more a certainty!?! Or would the men in white coats be knocking down my door?

Fortunately, around this time, I was directed to the book *Conversations with God* by Neale Donald Walsch. I read it cover to cover in record time. It answered many of the questions I had, as well as others I'd never even thought to ask. After reading a section, I'd ask, "Is that true?" and receive a clear yes to all my questions. Like Mr. Walsch, I was an average guy who'd made mistakes. I was both admired and disliked. I had an inner yet completely unconscious knowing that something else out there existed. I could feel it at times, but had no idea what it was or why it was there. This probably describes most, if not all, of us—which is exactly the point. If I can have this connection, so can all of you.

My fear of being seen as too different ran my life. I kept this connection hidden from others, including those who mattered the most—family, friends, and even girlfriends. Now, for all the world to read, at this time, I humbly apologize to all involved for my consciously chosen and totally fear-driven discretions.

But let me tell you: even with a clear channel to what I will now call by its literal nickname of *Source*, not all things are rosy, and in the beginning, when you are still a neophyte, it can be challenging to distinguish between actions suggested by Source and those presented as the only possible course by Ego.

Case in point. It was Ego that advised me to quit a well-paying and even cushy day job, after convincing me that all the things I needed would be handed to me now that I was on the spiritual path. Ego also let me believe I was taking time off to "find myself." I found myself alright—deep in debt! So there I was, unemployed, reading books on a park bench, and living on credit cards, and somehow able to communicate with something I doubted even existed not long before. It turns out that by listening to Ego not Source, I was getting a sorely needed lesson in humility. Ouch! It was a big wakeup call. Nothing would just be handed to me after all. Having this connection to Source was like reading a book—a really good book by a really great author; yet, I still had to do the necessary work. Spiritual growth can't be given, only earned.

Interestingly, as I did more muscle testing, as part of my work as a massage therapist in a chiropractor's office, my vibration began to rise. This enabled me to hear/feel the voice of Source pretty regularly and to begin to become a conduit for Source wisdom for others by sharing what I was intuiting. The words of Source seem to come through me in a particular way, depending on the situation or the client, and I have the odd sensation that it is not me, Dave, speaking; I am merely a channel. For example, I recall one lecture where I answered someone's question with one of the most brilliant responses ever! It was one of those catch phrases like *Do you live to eat or eat to live?* Yet I can't recall what was said or even what was asked. And when I ask Source about it I don't get an answer. Talk about a lesson in nonattachment!

Sometimes my all-too-human mind wants something right away and doesn't get it in its preferred way or time; yet, when I least expect it, something even greater finds its way toward me. Source teaches patience and likes to keep us on our toes. Another important element in working with Source that I have learned is that its use must always be ethical. Even though it's technically possible, I do not "energetically Google" others without their permission, which is a common fear that people have when they know that you are intuitive. *Do unto others* has been my credo. Whenever possible, I prefer to directly communicate with an individual as opposed to using a medium.

Another common misconception that people have when you channel Source is that things should flow easily. This is certainly what I always assumed. The Kabbalah, the mystic heart of Judaism, has some important things to say on this subject. It teaches that there are 10 layers of spiritual growth, and each of those has 10 layers as well. These layers are the 100 percentage points of awareness ranging from total ignorance to total enlightenment. To think we can leisurely skip through them is dubious at best. It's true that we come into this world with different levels of awareness, with different lessons to learn, but growth is a step-by-step process. Not until we're ready for the rewards that the higher levels promise will we experience them.

NOTE: *On the other side of every breakdown is a breakthrough.*

Many of us have already had our George Bailey moment, meaning we've been so down for so long that it begins to look like up. Less than 10 years ago I was jobless and still had rent, car payments, and credit card bills to pay just like many of you. Every job interview proved fruitless. During one particular interview for a job I knew I was overqualified for, the prospective employer sensed my lack of enthusiasm and actually asked me if I really wanted that job! My words could lie but my eyes gave me away. After a while of not doing much of anything, I felt worthless, morbidly lonely, and thought there was very little to live for. I had no girlfriend, no savings, no work, was thousands in debt, and such a bad liar I couldn't even trick anyone into hiring me. I was living a life of pretense. Everyone I knew thought I was nuts, lazy, stubborn, and arrogant, and could use counseling. I thought my life would get better on its own. It didn't. Denial had reared so loudly that I couldn't even hear it. Suddenly, fear, necessity, loneliness, and pain made me aware that I was despondent and in denial. I asked God for a sign.

> *There are times when we must sink to the bottom of our misery*
> *to understand truth, just as we must descend to the bottom of*
> *a well to see the stars in broad daylight.*
> —*VACLAV HAVEL, AUTHOR, FORMER CZECH REPUBLIC PRESIDENT*

Days had gone by and I forgot my request, and one afternoon on my driveway was a freshly broken egg with a baby pigeon in it. It was so tiny, so frail, so in need of care, yet apparently its mother had abandoned it after it fell from a nearby tree. I had no idea what to do. The pigeon was so helpless and made me see more clearly that I'd been helpless by my own accord for too long, too. Feeling no living creature should die on asphalt, I moved it onto the soft dirt under a nearby tree. A few hours later it passed away, and during the next few days it served as food for insects; shortly thereafter, its carcass had vanished completely.

This gift helped me see that all things and people have a purpose, whether alive or dead, and that I'd better find my purpose before it was too late. I stopped feeling sorry for myself, released all the worrying, and changed my attitude to one of thankfulness and compassion instead of the victim mentality that was keeping me down. At my next interview I was hired immediately, and it was only because my attitude had changed—my résumé and work experience were exactly the same! Overall, this experience made me realize how precious and temporary life is, and that any life can end at any moment. Oddly enough it wasn't death that frightened me. No, my worst fear, the one I felt strongest when imagining my own passing, was living in mediocrity not having shared all my gifts.

> *A person's life purpose is nothing more than to rediscover,*
> *through the detours of art, or love, or passionate work,*
> *those one or two images in the presence of which that*
> *person's heart first opened.*
> —*ALBERT CAMUS, AUTHOR*

CHAPTER 1

Unlocking the Cause of Ill Health

*My doctor gave me six months to live, but when I couldn't
pay the bill, he gave me six months more.*
—*WOODY ALLEN, COMEDIAN AND FILMMAKER*

After a few years as a New York state–licensed massage therapist (LMT), during which I had no concern about or belief in the intangibles (energy, meridians, past lives, and so on), some clients began telling me what they were "seeing" when their muscles were being worked on. Some said they could see flashbacks to when they were young. Some of these visions seemed to come from another time altogether. I certainly had my doubts, but I wondered how many were having similar visions and didn't say anything, perhaps thinking that their experience was too weird to mention. I later learned that *where* or *why* or even *if* any of these events actually happened was irrelevant. The important message was that the memory was somehow stored in their body and it was merely being triggered by whatever we were doing. The memories could have been real, made up, or even from a dream, and although I really didn't want to believe it, while working with and getting to know my clients, a connection between the mind and body became very apparent.

It became so obvious to me that certain patterns of thought created certain types of pain that eventually I was able to make a reference map of what I was finding. A reflexology chart shows you how you can apply pressure to a certain point of the foot and doing so can affect another location in the body. Traditional Chinese Medicine (TCM), which has been around for 5,000 years, also uses certain points distant from the area being worked on. It is equally clear that areas of pain in the body hold emotional connections that definitely began elsewhere. Memories and emotions are thoughts, and all thoughts mobilize energy. Energy when focused with enough intensity and/or frequency of thought is what creates your individual reality. Energy that is repressed has to go somewhere, and where it goes— initially at least—is to your muscles. Continued repression of this energy creates stiffness and pain. Further repression creates more systemic—or what is called more serious—pain and illness. And so began the realization that there is more to health and illness than our traditional healthcare system is aware of.

How do I know this for sure? Because when I intuit that someone has a particular issue, say anger against his father, and that individual's pain goes away without me physically touching that individual when all other attempts—physical or mental—have failed, that repeated success dictates firm belief.

Sometimes, while I'm working with someone's neck or back pain on their left side, they will say that it has mysteriously moved to the right side. If pain were physical only, such as a muscle or tendon tear, how can the pain move from one side to the other? It doesn't. That individual is simply becoming aware of the emotional cause of his pain. Until then, his mind had blocked out what was causing the pain. Harmful thought patterns are stored inside the body and do not dissipate on their own. It takes a direct and conscious approach to eliminate them. By understanding the cause from a larger, more inclusive and holistic perspective, you are more able to prevent and release the pain—permanently.

Healing with Source, Example No. 1

"I've had sciatica with varying amounts of pain, ranging from moderate to excruciating. For 40 years I've had this [discomfort], and some days I was unable to walk. In one session with David, I experienced about an 80 percent reduction in pain and by the next day—and ever since then—I have been completely pain-free."

—NINA P., TAROT CARD READER

Nina realized the various treatments she'd been following were only intermittently helpful. During that 40-year period, there were some moments of pain-free living, but they were sporadic at best. **I asked her *when* the pain would occur.** She replied, "while standing up." Upon hearing this, I shared what I heard intuitively, that she does not have sciatica. Her reaction, of course, was confusion and doubt because for 40 years she'd been told that she did have sciatica.

What do we know about sciatica?

Sciatica is pain, tingling, or numbness produced by an irritation of the sciatic nerve. The sciatic nerve is formed by the nerve roots coming out of the spinal cord into the lower back. Branches of the sciatic nerve extend through the buttocks and down the back of each leg to the ankle and foot. What causes sciatica? The most common cause of sciatica is a bulging or ruptured disc (herniated disc) in the spine pressing against the sciatic nerve… Branches of the sciatic nerve extend through the buttocks and down the back of each leg to the ankle and foot .[1]

The diagnoses, treatments, and prognoses Nina received didn't work because none of them determined or addressed the hidden causes of a bulging or ruptured disc. Nor is it clear what the presence of a bulging or herniated disc has to do with pain .[2] According to a study done by the George Washington University Medical Center,[3] almost one third of *asymptomatic* (not in pain) MRI recipients had an "identifiable abnormality of a disc or of the spinal canal." Therefore, the presence of herniated discs has little to do with the amount of pain someone is experiencing.

Even so, a medical doctor's diagnosis of sciatica (also called *piriformis syndrome*) might include a recommendation of physical therapy and medication, and they will often predict a year's recovery time, which is often the case. Oh, how right they are! A chiropractor might diagnose this pain as *vertebral subluxations* and recommend spinal adjustments, usually starting out at three times per week and very gradually decreasing that amount while predicting recovery at six to eight months—and it often takes that long! Right again! An acupuncturist may diagnose this symptom as an imbalance in the gall bladder meridian (the acupoint being GB-30, which is a warehouse for anger), and recommend two to three treatments per week for two to three months. Once again, correct!

The length of time for the patient to recover will vary. A practitioner will see what they have been trained to see and act accordingly. Words have power, and by diagnosing this type of pain as sciatica/piriformis syndrome, a vertebral subluxation, or even a gall bladder meridian imbalance, the patient will be most amenable to the commonly accepted understanding and prognosis associated with each. Because the patient believes these well-meaning practitioners, the patient's healing time will usually be close to their prediction. I, however, call it "a temporary misalignment in the quantum field of pure potentiality," or more simply, an opportunity to discover and release the hidden cause.

I told Nina that because she believed her doctors, she would most likely be helped in both the amount of pain relief and time that these practitioners thought possible.

---

1 http://www.webmd.com/hw/back_pain/tp22230.asp

2 http://clinicaltrials.gov/ct/gui/show/NCT00011739;jsessionid=D5F8C3020C6F2A1B781F713A5 AC96831?order=5 A Prospective Cohort Study of MRI Abnormalities and Back Pain Risk: Low back pain is a frequent cause of disability and a common reason for outpatient care in veterans. Magnetic resonance imaging (MRI) of the lower back often reveals abnormalities, which may be used to justify expensive and invasive therapy, such as surgery. Yet the link between MRI abnormalities and the risk of developing clinically significant back pain is far from clear.

3 http://www.ncbi.nlm.nih.gov/entrez/query.fcgi?cmd=Retrieve&db=PubMed&dopt=Abstract& list_uids=11568190

Unfortunately for Nina, it was a much longer period of time than they predicted or hoped for. Therefore, a change in perspective was needed. Because she only experienced this pain while standing up, I shared what I heard intuitively from Source, that she had a "standing up" problem and not sciatica!

I asked her what the words "standing up" meant to her. She said it was about taking responsibility. We talked about that for a few minutes and looked into what, or more accurately, who, she was feeling responsible for. It turned out that she was feeling responsible for her 40-year-old daughter. While some level of responsibility can be appreciated, ultimately, her daughter had to live her own life. A parent can guide a child, but at some point, the "energetic cord of responsibility" must be cut. We concluded that this behavior was not what she wished to experience—that her daughter had to learn her own lessons.

No matter how much one cares for one's child, no one is responsible for the path of another's soul. When Nina accepted this new perspective, we did some Healing with Source energy work. After just a few minutes, I felt a shift and asked her to stand up. At that point, she claimed to have experienced an 80 percent reduction in pain. When I saw her a few months later, she said that within a day of her last and only visit—and up until that point—she was living pain-free.

When you picked up this book, you probably already knew, or were at least hoping to have confirmed, that what is conventionally thought to be the cause of pain or illness is merely the tip of the iceberg. To date, Western medicine rarely takes into account the connections among mind, spirit, and body in treating the physical body. This methodology clearly leaves millions of people with chronic pain, most of whom depend on drugs to get them through the day or are overly dependent on well-meaning healthcare practitioners. If these medications and practitioners are needed, then be thankful they are there. Use whatever is necessary to better your life, but know that in most cases, what we are usually hoping for, and therefore get, is temporary pain management.

Our remedies oft in ourselves do lie.
—*SHAKESPEARE, PLAYWRIGHT AND POET*

Many medications merely mask the symptoms. They trick your brain into thinking you are better by dulling your perception of the symptoms. In reality, the root cause of your symptoms is still there making things worse. That's like cutting the wires of a fire alarm because the ringing is annoying: by the time you see the fire, it's too late. Rarely—if ever—does utilizing medication lead to long-term healing; more often what occurs, by design, is a temporary elimination of the symptoms. It is clear that while we look beyond ourselves for the causes of pain and illness, true healing is better begun by looking inward. We need to replace this telescopic ideology with that of an electron microscope!

"Monica" believed solely in the tangible, Western medical paradigm, which told her she needed shoulder surgery. Afterward, she was told to do rehabilitative exercises, but her range of motion was limited due to the nonelasticity of her deltoid muscle. The muscle could only go so far without sensations of pain being sent to and from the brain. In this case, the pain was a gift—a signal that only X amount, say three inches, of movement was possible. Because she needed to do the exercises and couldn't, her doctor recommended taking a pain reliever. All this did was to prevent her from perceiving at what point her muscles were being stretched beyond the three inches, her current edge. There was no sensation of pain—no warning system in her conscious awareness letting her know how far she should move. Like a rubber band, a muscle can only stretch so far without damage. Because of the insular paradigm presented by her doctor and the numbing effects of the "pain reliever," her predicted two-month recovery took almost a year.

Repressed emotions such as anger can lead to muscle pain and stiffness, usually and initially in the neck and/or upper back. This can lead to headaches because nerve, blood, and oxygen flow to the brain are reduced. Given that information, one could say that headaches are caused by muscular tightness in the neck area and the muscles, therefore, need to be relaxed. True—to a point.

All the temporary cures in the world can make you feel better, but the repressed emotion that caused the muscle tightness to begin with will still be there. This is why people with migraine headaches, for example, continue to experience pain and receive little help from body-only medicine, be it dentistry, physical therapy, medication, osteopathy, medication, chiropractic, acupuncture, or even massage, although the latter would make the most sense. Of course, there are some instances where any or all of these are seemingly effective, but it is lengthy and costly, and still doesn't get to the root of the problem.

The first problem for all of us… is not to learn, but to unlearn.
—*GLORIA STEINEM, EDITOR*

Continually repressed anger over longer periods of time can manifest in other areas. According to TCM, the gall bladder and liver are the internal organs where anger can be held. It is easy to look at that and say, "But what about Uncle Fred? Isn't his liver damage a result of his drinking?" Yes it can be, and you can operate on the liver or even perform a transplant, but without getting to the source of his liver problem, what are the chances of full healing? If not addressed, the emotional causes will in time affect his new liver as well. Beyond obvious physical incompatibilities, this is often termed *rejection*. It is a cycle that needs to be looked at as a whole. Is Uncle Fred's problem his drinking? If you said yes, you are half right, but drinking alcohol is a symptom, not a cause. The cause can be revealed by asking, *Why he is drinking in the first place?* We can then ask, *What emotional pain is being repressed so often and so intensely that it is leading Uncle Fred to drink?*

If the causal energy is directly addressed either during or after Uncle Fred's surgery, his liver transplant will be more effective! If it is found before the operation, he may be able to avoid the surgery. If it is discovered earlier than that, maybe he can avoid his headaches. If it is seen even earlier, maybe he can avoid the neck pain. If it is discovered even before that, maybe Uncle Fred would be able to recognize the anger and release it before any damage occurs. If it were observed before that, that is if Uncle Fred had been taught and then applied anger management skills, none of this would even matter. We might call this the anti-domino effect, a healthy reversal of what usually happens in Western medicine.

Healing with Source, Example No. 2

"Alex" said he had terrible reactions to warm climates. He said it seemed like every time he went away, he'd wind up with intestinal discomfort. One could easily say it may have been the food or water, but I was guided to ask him the following questions (in boldface):

> **"Where have you gone recently that made these symptoms develop?"**
> "Florida."
> **"Have you gone to the Caribbean, or Bermuda?"**
> "Yes, of course."
> **"And do these symptoms develop there, too?"**
> "Well, actually, no. No, they don't."
> **"So what's in Florida that isn't in these other places?"**
> Alex smiled as if we'd hit the nail on the head. "My parents!"

> *"He who asks a question is a fool for five minutes;*
> *he who does not ask a question remains a fool forever."*
> —*CHINESE PROVERB*

By asking Nina the right questions, I helped her reduce and then eliminate pain that she was calling sciatica because it only occurred during a certain movement—standing up. "Alex" got to the root of his quandary by answering some questions that hadn't yet been asked elsewhere. Solely by posing the right questions and avoiding drawing incorrect or premature conclusions, we arrived at the hidden cause of his symptoms. By addressing his relationship with his parents, we could minimize his visceral reactions to them.

So, how do we avoid drawing incorrect conclusions? By writing with the eraser side of the pencil! Your thoughts and perspectives are a creative flow, constantly changing in response to conditions, and therefore always able to shift. Your whole being is a manifestation of what you are creating inside you moment to moment. *So it follows that your current state of health or illness is the impermanent end result of your creative beliefs.* We all know someone who feared having a particular pain or illness who ended up with that exact pain or illness. Fear is a powerful creative force. Your body will always follow your thoughts—good, bad, or indifferent to what you say you really want.

Early on in my career as a massage therapist, I got to know many clients well and soon realized that those who complained a lot had tighter muscles than those who were generally more content. While it is typical to say their frustration about their muscular tightness is because of their physical condition, experience has taught me it is actually the reverse! Their muscles are a direct result of all the emotional "poison" they've created. This emotional poison is the residue of years of emotional turmoil that has accumulated in their bodies. Take, for example, a man who attended a Healing with Source class I held a few years ago:

For many years, "Burt" couldn't turn his head to the right. He'd seen every specialist there was and still no one could help him. I immediately picked up that he held a lot of anger in his neck muscles, especially toward his son. I shared my observation with him, and he agreed that he did have a lot of anger toward his son, but never made the connection between that anger and his neck pain. Burt then asked what he should do.

I reminded him that if the mind and body are connected, and that he's had this pain for all this time and no one could help him, it was time to make better choices—to help himself. I told him the answer was quite simple and so close to him he couldn't even see it. He had to smooth out whatever differences he had with his son—with a professional mediator, if need be. His reaction was indignation at best. Burt was determined to take this anger with him to the grave and to hold his son responsible.

While that may have seemed right to Burt—that it's okay to be angry with another person—I took this opportunity to point out the choice between being loving and being right. "Burt, you cannot be both. You've been living this way for how long? And it still hasn't worked." Why? Because being right is a function of Ego, and Ego thrives on controversy, wanting to prove itself right. Unfortunately, this is often done at the expense of another individual, for if one person has to be right, he or she will make another person wrong just to prove a point. The obvious drawback is that few people want to be told they're wrong—even if they are! The recipient of this perceived verbal onslaught is quite naturally repelled from its source and drawn to defend himself, and no one can win a war that does not need to be fought!

I could almost see and feel Burt's whole life story in each line on his withered face. He told me, "My father was tough and made a man out of me, and I tried to do that with my son, too, and he's rejected everything I've ever told him."

I then shared that children do not want to be told what to do. Telling a child (or even an adult) what to do only pushes the child away and makes the young person reject what they're being told by even the most well-meaning parent—no matter how good the advice may be. Children would rather be listened to than spoken to! This doesn't mean that a parent shouldn't guide the child, but more from the perspective of making it clear that there are consequences to all choices. Once a child knows WHY something is required and knows he or she will be supported in their decisions, he or she will often make the best choice. But if a child is ordered to clean his room or to pursue a high-status job "because I said so" or because "everyone else is doing it," it won't make any sense to that young person and will only result in rebellion.

"On the other hand, to love unconditionally is a choice of the heart," I continued. "The heart wants peace and harmony. Using the heart to make choices (as opposed to Ego) and looking at things with a much wider lens can only lead to happiness in the long run."

I asked Burt if he understood. He said yes, he did. I then asked: "Are you ready to have that long-awaited conversation with your son now? Are you ready to accept his choices, even if you don't agree with them?" He then went back into a tirade of blame. "But my son did this… ! My son said that… ! Why should I… ? Yada, yada…"

I let him vent for a bit and, when he calmed down I reiterated, "So, you're saying that you understood everything I said, and that it even makes sense to you, yet you still refuse to even try to smooth things out?" Maybe Burt's need to live in a world where things are labeled either right or wrong was challenged and he saw how poor his choices were, because at the break he quietly left. Like a good parent, I can only guide someone to another truth and accept them unconditionally; what they do after that is their choice.

Those who are emotionally inflexible will usually have muscles that are physically inflexible. Those who are stubborn will have muscles that do not want to give in to treatment. Those harboring repressed anger will continue to live in a painful, unpleasant way, and their muscles will pay the price for their stubbornness. Their sessions, if they are even willing to participate, will likely be longer and more intense. They will often believe that deep, physical work is needed because they've experienced temporary relief in the past from that type of work. In the short term, this makes a lot of sense as endorphins are released and the perception is that the pain is lessened, but they still have the problem and always will if the other factors are not addressed. You cannot reverse anything using the same energy that created it, and deep tissue work is too reminiscent of the causal factors (pain) for healing to occur.

> NOTE: *Stubbornness is a function of Ego—the individual life force within you. Ego perceives spiritual growth to be the death of itself and will fight to survive.*

People will first create their pain, then continue to create situations that keep their pain intact. Some people define themselves by their pain; they like to complain about something because it hooks the attention of others. Not you, of course, but the other guy. Misery seems to live up to its reputation and loves the company. Those individuals are less likely to see an improvement in their condition because the rewards of getting attention outweigh the benefits of healing.

For example: How many people do you know who when referring to their pain or illness have said that they can live with it or that it's meant to be? Sorry, there is no preordained reason to accept a life of suffering. Such thinking comes from a defeatist mind-set. As a result, there is no real chance of healing anything.

What is mind?
No matter.
What is matter?
Never mind.

You've heard people say they hold their stress and tension in their neck and shoulders. So, why is it so odd to hear that we hold anger in our lower back? Or grief in our upper chest? It is unusual only because we weren't taught that there is a mind-body connection—that they are different aspects of us but they are not related, especially in matters of maintaining health.

You've experienced physical symptoms within seconds of particular thoughts. Crying, laughing, and even walking are end results of thoughts. When you watch a sad scene in a movie you may begin to cry. Sometimes this is accompanied by a "lump in your throat." If you continue to experience (create) the "lump in the throat," you may soon experience (cause) a runny nose. If you continue to experience (create) the runny nose, you may create intestinal discomfort. All of these symptoms are manifestations of thoughts. You saw something that wasn't even real and perceived it as sad, and the physical manifestations, or symptoms, followed immediately.

You are driving and another vehicle seems to be heading toward you at high speed. You perceive this as a dangerous situation, and your body immediately goes into *fight or flight*. This is a sympathetic nervous system response, an ancient gift designed to protect us from a perceived enemy or predator. It allows us to quickly and efficiently act upon a situation to minimize or eliminate the possibility of danger. First, you will produce adrenaline in your adrenal glands and sweat profusely within milliseconds of the initial perception! Blood is shunted to specific areas based on your decision to fight or take flight or freeze, and breathing is altered to become quicker and shallow during sympathetic activation versus deep and relaxed during the parasympathetic response, often called the "relaxation or rest-and-restore response." Again, you saw or felt something that was interpreted as dangerous, and the physical manifestations followed immediately!

A few years ago, I was cut off when exiting a New York City subway train. Stopped midstride, my right leg fell into the gap between the subway car and the platform, and I must have somehow managed to push myself out quickly. I say *must have somehow* because I don't remember any of it. This get-out-of-danger, unconscious reaction was an example of the primitive fight-or-flight response. Something deep within my brain took over faster than my ability to process what had happened! In fact, if I didn't have scars all along my right leg and rips in the pants, I'd never have believed it happened.

Your body reacts to every thought. Safety or, at minimum, homeostasis/balance is its prime directive. What would happen if, for example, you were experiencing a strong emotion over a considerably longer period of time? What happens if you are angry and do not deal with it right away, but repress it? What do you think happens when someone dies and you do not fully grieve? What happens when fear is kept locked within? Thoughts are energy that is concentrated by intention, and energy sets into motion the transformation or even the creation of matter. Where else would all of this creative energy manifest itself if it is not released? It has to go somewhere.

NOTE: *Externally directed anger is like taking poison and expecting it to kill the other person.*

Perhaps you are in a relationship and your partner is unfaithful. As a child, perhaps you felt neglected or were abused. Perhaps you are disrespected at work or by your peers. It's natural to feel hurt. In time, resentment builds up inside you. Anger then follows. Your breath shortens. Your neck muscles tighten. You think about revenge. You may even hope for something bad to happen to the person you perceive as the perpetrator. Your breathing becomes shallow because your mind already is. It is not your fault, you think:

you were conditioned into believing your current reality. But this version of reality needs an adjustment. To be healthy, you need to change your perspective from victim to victor.

Don't Touch My Hands!

A great place to begin reversing our perspective on manifestations of pain and illness in the body is to take a simple idea, usually put forward as truth, that germs spread through hand-to-hand contact and to reconsider its merits. We're told that germs spread through contact with contaminated surfaces and lead to what we've been taught to believe is the common cold. And yet it is entirely possible, and even accepted by Western medicine, that two persons can come into contact with the same pathogen, or germ that causes disease, and only one of them will get sick. This has even been proven with much more serious alleged causes of illness; HIV is not always transferred (manifested) between partners where one is infected. In either case, if it was only the pathogen responsible for illness, *everyone* exposed to it would have contracted it!

What makes one person immune and another succumb to the same pathogens? This is the question we should be asking ourselves—not spending inordinate amounts of time on what to do *after* something is contracted. Louis Pasteur, who discovered microscopic pathogens and spent much of his life convincing others they were real and at fault for many illnesses, in his later years concluded, "The germ is nothing; the terrain is all."

This "terrain" is our emotional state. Our emotions and state of mind affect our immune system. Most disease conditions manifest themselves as a result of a weakened immune system. Self-hatred, irritability, stress, judging, nonacceptance, or resistance to what is both within and outside us will weaken our immune system. Marianne Williamson, author of *A Return to Love* and other spiritual books, has said that if we spoke to others the way we speak to ourselves, we'd have no friends. In fact, if verbal self-attacks are something you do more often than not, and words have energy and energy alters matter, your immune system's strength will be weakened. It may even attack itself.

The person who always feels he or she will get sick by participating in a given activity will usually get sick performing that activity. Yet not everyone who performs that activity gets sick. John feels that eating fast will cause him to experience diarrhea; therefore, it often does. Stephen can eat the same food in the same amount of time and not be adversely affected. Shyler will not eat red meat because she feels that it will be difficult to digest and she will feel "heavy" afterward. Tonya will eat a cheeseburger with all the fixings and french fries, and not only enjoy it but still feel healthy without feeling heavy or lethargic. Marc will avoid touching handles because he feels he will contract germs and get sick because that's what he was taught—that germs are spread by hand-to-germ contact and cause sickness if his hands then touch a mucous membrane like the eyes or nose. Yet

Laura will grab the handle and then touch her mucous membranes and not succumb to illness. We have our own ideas about what will get us sick solely as a result of believing what we have been told. What would happen if we consciously changed that belief?

Deciding to change your mind may be the easiest part of the equation; changing your mind and believing you have actually done so may be a bit more difficult.

If we truly believe we will not get sick by touching door handles or feel lethargic after eating a cheeseburger with all the fixings, then, indeed, we will not experience sickness or lethargy. This is the power of the mind. After reading Eric Schlosser's bestseller *Fast Food Nation*, which illuminates the awful and unsanitary conditions behind the meat industry, I decided to eliminate burgers from my diet. One day I gave in to an old habit and ordered a burger. The first bite felt like a brick moving slowly down my throat and digestive tract and actually caused intense pain! Instantly worried and about to panic big time, I was relieved when about 20 seconds later I actually threw up. The burger in itself was no different from countless others I'd eaten before. Only my perspective on it had changed!

Any doubts we are having consciously or otherwise will reduce the efficiency of the process, so it is best to start out small, working with what you believe is possible before doing anything drastic. There are those who have believed they could fly but could not, because there are some forces that are too great to alter at this stage of our evolution. Very few have walked on water, yet thousands (myself included) have walked across a bed of hot coals. I've seen people walk on broken pieces of glass, and even saw two beloved friends bend a rebar with their throats. Please do not try any of these at home or anywhere else based on these statements alone; I mention these examples only to show you that just because you have yet to do something doesn't mean that with proper training it can't be done. As with the four-minute mile, no one believed it was possible until Roger Bannister actually did it. And then many followed.

CHAPTER 2

The Hidden Causes of Pain and Illness

Give light, and the darkness will disappear of itself.
—*ERASMUS, HUMANIST AND THEOLOGIAN*

It should be pretty clear by now that our thoughts and our ways of doing and being directly correlate with our physical symptoms and conditions. While external factors such as genetic and environmental conditions have an undeniable influence, we have a lot more power to create our own reality than we realize. That resurgence of personal power exists for a very good reason, which we'll discuss later.

When I work with individual clients and groups, the most frequent request I get is to give details on the connections between specific thought patterns and pains or illness. While I'd never presume to know your entire life just from hearing about your symptoms, the commonalities are too universal to omit. There are always exceptions. The following are brief explanations of some of the most common causes and symptoms; more details follow. Like everything in this book, take what resonates and simply discard the rest.

Unilateral Upper Back Pain

Alfred lent $1,000 to his best friend Bernie. Bernie agreed to pay Alfred back in four months but didn't follow through on his commitment. Alfred began to wonder if he would ever see that money again. He felt a bit angry, but decided not to say anything. Within a few weeks of the payback date, he felt a stabbing sensation in his upper back. As time went on, he got angrier and still didn't say anything. Alfred, quite naturally, felt he'd been stabbed in the back.

What Alfred didn't know is that by feeling he'd been stabbed in the back, he had actually manifested the pain in his upper back between the scapula and spine. In fact, this is where most physical stabbings occur, and it is also where mental stabbings are

31

pictured. Such is the power of the mind-body connection: what you see, hear, or feel becomes real!

✪ Reclaim your birthright of joy!

Alfred's pain was on the right side, which in TCM is called the *yang* (masculine) side. This is one of your body's ways of symbolically telling you what's wrong and who needs to be forgiven! If it were on the left, the *yin* side, the anger would be toward feminine energy. Does this sound odd? Hey, I don't make the rules, I just channel them. Note that masculine energy does not solely mean male energy nor is feminine energy limited to the female; it merely describes traditional characteristics of each. Just as black and white flow seamlessly together into a circle to create the eternal yin-yang symbol, we all have both feminine and masculine energy within us, but usually one predominates. The stabbing pain in Alfred's upper back got worse when he thought about his best friend's betrayal, but he put it down to sleeping poorly, overdoing it at the gym, or bad posture, having been taught to look outside himself for answers. As Alfred's anger overcame him, the pain only got stronger.

On the six-month anniversary of the loan, which also happened to be Alfred's 40th birthday, Bernie showed up at Alfred's workplace and offered to pay for lunch. Alfred figured he'd get back about $20 worth of food from his $1,000 and said okay. As he took his first bite, Bernie presented Alfred with a check for $1,500 saying, "Remember that investment I was telling you about? The one that you didn't care to invest in. Well, I thought it was too good to pass up and I knew we'd all make a killing, so I invested your $1,000 for you! So Happy Birthday, and congratulations on a wise investment!"

Here you have the same situation with two completely different perspectives. From his point of view, Bernie did something completely innocent, while Alfred spent the whole six months being angry and feeling like he'd been stabbed in the back. He had been—only it was he who had done the stabbing!

Not all situations will work themselves out so clearly, but this is an example of how two different realities can be constructed around the same event and how the subsequent anger can cause physical pain. If you are unwilling or unable to peacefully converse with the person you feel has victimized you, try working it out on your own. Even writing them a letter that you never send can be helpful. What have you go to lose, except for your old ways of being that no longer serve you?

How About Neck Pain?

When we perceive a situation as stressful, our breathing is altered to utilize the secondary breathing muscles; our bodies want to get air quicker as opposed to deeper. The diaphragm, the primary breathing muscle during relaxed periods, is utilized only minimally in these situations. The secondary breathing muscles located in the neck elevate the ribcage creating a vacuum whereby you can breathe. If they are used as primary breathing muscles for too long, they can become overused, causing the muscles to tighten and minimize blood and oxygen flow. This, in turn, creates sensations of pain and stiffness, and eventually headaches. And it is all because we perceived something as stressful.

Energetically, the stress held in the neck muscles often means we are too hard on ourselves. Self-judgment and self-criticism create stress and shorten the breath.

If the pain in the neck is on one side only, you are harboring anger toward someone other than yourself. These unilateral pains are usually manifested in the muscles that rotate the head left or right. The person you are blaming has been perceived by you as "a pain in the neck," and because of the creative power of thoughts you will have created a pain in your neck! The same process is at play with a "pain in the butt," a condition some people refer to as sciatica. Words create our reality, and everything is related to our thoughts—even metaphorically.

Lower Back, Knee, Ankle, and Arch of the Foot Pains

"I had been living with severe pain in my knee and hip for a couple of years. I tried guided imagery and hypnosis with a medical doctor, acupuncture (which usually is effective for my arthritis, but not in this case), and pain medication, all to no avail. I knew the pain was a mind-body problem relating to unresolved family issues, but it's difficult to resolve conflicts when the people involved have passed on. Nevertheless, that's what we accomplished in only five sessions. With deep breathing exercises and Dave's hands-on manipulation, Dave talked me through the process of letting go, forever, of old hurts that serve no purpose. To my relief, literally and figuratively, the old pain has not resurfaced in the subsequent six years. I've also attended Dave's Healing Circles a few times every year to remind me to stay focused in the present and to surround myself with the positive energy of the Healing Circle itself. Thank you Dave!"

—*ANGIE, SECRETARY, NEW YORK CITY*

The lower back, knees, ankles, and arches of the feet are areas that support you. Pain in these areas can be caused by lack of support either for you from others or from you toward others. Intense emotion gets locked in these areas because of the support you feel you haven't been given but thought you deserved, or anger you've created because you are supporting someone else who perhaps does not show their appreciation.

If you feel you were not given the support you deserve, don't be surprised that if the people you perceive to have done that were asked the same question, they'd feel you weren't supportive of them! Step away from your own feelings and realize this person has a support issue as well. By doing so, you will have a better understanding of what is happening. If someone fails to show appreciation for the support you are giving them, the pain you feel may be due to your anger at them or yourself because you let it happen that way. Sensing a pattern yet?

Also, the lower back tends to hold longer-standing emotions, such as anger toward a family member. These can be relatively more difficult to reverse, but it is possible. By reprocessing the event that caused the anger and releasing the energy either on your own or with a practitioner, lower back pain can become a thing of the past.

Allergies and Other Breathing Ailments, Elimination Problems, Obesity, and Depression

Don't be dismayed at goodbyes; a farewell is necessary before you can meet again.
And meeting again, after moments or lifetimes, is certain for those who are friends.
—RICHARD BACH, AUTHOR

Repressed grief can cause a host of physical ailments: allergies, bronchial problems, elimination problems, skin eruptions, obesity, and even depression. It is important to understand the grief process fully to utilize it as it was meant to be used. It is a built-in system for dealing with loss in a healthy way. More on this later.

Food Allergies

These are often the result of childhood control issues made manifest. Most of my clients who present with food allergies had parents who tried to control them via reward and punishment with food. How many of you can relate to the line spoken angrily on Pink Floyd's *The Wall* CD: "If you don't eat your meat, you can't have any pudding! How can you have any pudding if you don't eat your meat!?" I've seen people minimize and even reverse their food allergy just by following the Five Steps to Health! More on this later.

Inflexibility in Muscles and Joints

If you have stiffness or pain in your joints, you have a flexibility problem, not a joint problem. You have been inflexible in your ways of thought! It may have started out as soreness or a pulled muscle, but you were most likely unaware of why the soreness or pulled muscle happened. You may have experienced temporary pain reduction from medical treatment, but without addressing the cause, the problems return. They either come back as a more severe version of what you already experienced, or they assisted in creating a pain elsewhere in a chain reaction of unconscious, postural compensation. For example, if pain were in your right knee and you had to adjust your walk, the left knee may compensate and be overused. The result is two problematic knees, but the hidden cause is still in the right knee.

It's time to recognize your stubbornness has hampered your job, or a relationship, or even your creativity. Dig deeply within and ask yourself if this uncompromising behavior is serving you. If yes, then have a nice day. If no, then it is time to figure out why you have been so stubborn.

Stubbornness is a thought process left over from all the times we wanted to get our way but didn't. This is the mind of our inner three-year-old whose mind-set is still running—and perhaps even ruining—our lives. It is time to re-create yourself anew with this new awareness in each moment called NOW.

Of Course, There Are Movement Pains

As mentioned earlier, if you have a pain in your lower back but only feel it when you are standing up, you do not have a lower back problem, you very likely have a "standing up" problem! You can treat your lower back all you wish and with any modality you feel is beneficial, but you will not experience true, permanent healing because your back pain when standing is a symptom, and not a cause. Ask yourself what "standing up" means to you. Just as the feeling of being stabbed in the back manifests in upper back pain, lower-back pain serves as another metaphor for an issue in your life. Standing up could mean taking responsibility, being recognized, standing up for yourself, harboring issues around being respected, taking a stand on something. The list could go on.

Shoulder Pain or Pain When Raising Your Arm Overhead

If you feel pain when you raise your arm above your head, this too can be a manifestation of any random thoughts already within you that are associated with this movement. An inability to easily raise your hand may indicate acknowledgment issues or anger at a schoolteacher. You have to figure out what it means to you, but you can be assured that some metaphorical connection exists. Do you feel you have the weight of the world on your shoulders? Or have you for too long been someone else's shoulder to cry on?

S- and C-Shaped Spinal Curves (Scoliosis)

If tight muscles are reacting from intense repressed anger as a child, it can alter the skeletal system during the formative years. Intense unilateral anger (left/feminine – right/masculine) if not addressed early enough will often cause what is called scoliosis—a C-shaped curve in the spine. In some instances, this will self-compensate and create an S-shaped curve. Perhaps later in life, the physical manifestations of spinal deformities may be too ingrained for rapid healing, but the painful symptoms associated with them can certainly be reduced. Then, as time goes on, perhaps a shift in the skeletal system may occur. Be patient, not a patient.

Cold Hands and Feet

Persons with cold hands and feet are quick to say they have a circulation problem, even if their exercise routine is the same as that of another person with warm hands and feet. They are also quick to blame low blood pressure, but the cause of either the poor circulation or the low blood pressure has yet to be identified! By just saying you have poor circulation or low blood pressure, you are doing nothing to alleviate the symptoms. You are giving in to a diagnosis, an interpretation of a given set of information based on other people's symptoms. By accepting this, you define yourself as a victim of its characteristics and lose the opportunity to improve your situation by staying open to its causes and remedies. Eventually, cold hands and feet can become so uncomfortable that you may find yourself being labeled as having Reynard's disease, for which in Western medicine there is not only no cure but no explanation of the cause.

When you are in a situation that your body perceives as stressful, it will automatically go into a sympathetic fight-or-flight nervous system protective response, or if the danger is so great that action of any kind is deemed hopeless, an extreme parasympathetic response that will lead to freezing, or playing dead. When you perceive something as dangerous enough to run away from, adrenaline is automatically secreted by your adrenal glands and blood is diverted to leg muscles to prepare you to get out of harm's way. When your body decides to fight, meaning it wishes to deal with the perceived threat head on, blood will be shunted to the inner organs to protect those organs that you cannot live without. It is possible to live without legs, but not without many of your internal organs. In the case of extreme stress overload, where neither response is deemed appropriate, the body may go into a complete freeze, the most primitive of the reactions. All of this happens solely because your mind perceives a situation as stressful!

On a purely physical level, if you are in this fight mode for too long, what do you think will happen? You will have less blood going into your extremities and will end up with—you guessed it—cold hands and cold feet.

Yawning and Lethargy

Though not a pain, illness, or malady, it is accepted that a yawn is an end result of being tired. Granted this may be true, but what causes tiredness?

You are tired when you are stagnant in mind, thoughts, or body. Stagnation creates a larger need for air in the body. So, yawning is a wakeup call to get up and do something! You will never see an athlete yawn in mid-performance. Our perception of "tired" has been twisted; we think it is only related to not getting enough sleep. While this can be a factor, it should be noted that the happiest people—those whose lives are full with fun, learning, and love—need much less sleep than others. They aren't happy *because* of this lack of a need to sleep; it's more that they are happy by choice and, therefore, need less sleep. They wish to get up early and take advantage of all the day has to offer. Their activity, whether mental, physical, or spiritual keeps them awake. You yawn because your body needs to get air deep into your lungs. You yawn to get the diaphragm working again. You yawn because you have been too stagnant. I'm yawning just writing about it!

The animal kingdom can be used as inspiration here. What is the first thing your dog does when he awakes? He gets his energy and blood flowing, right? If he had a yoga mat, you'd describe these motions as downward dog, followed by upward dog, and then a shake! (I wonder why yogis exclude the shake in the sun salutation series.) Try it. Be like a dog and wag your tail; it's fun and healthy!

You only lose energy when life becomes dull in your mind.
Your mind gets bored and, therefore, tired of doing nothing.
Get interested in something! Get absolutely enthralled in something!
Get out of yourself! Be somebody! Do something.
The more you lose yourself in something bigger than yourself,
the more energy you will have.
—*NORMAN VINCENT PEALE, AUTHOR*

Numerous disempowering labels such as chronic fatigue are given to people who have low energy. Little to none of it is ultimately true. High energy levels are an end result of movement, not conservation. (Please don't use this as permission to overdo it; use uncommon sense!) Energy is always in motion. How can you conserve and try to hold still that which cannot be still by its very nature? You might as well tell the scorpion not to sting its prey. Even if it understood English, it would scoff at the thought!

Throat, Voice, and Thyroid Problems

Sore throats, mucous build-up/continual throat clearing, voice difficulties, larynx problems, thyroid issues, and more are end results of energetic blockages in the throat chakra. As the throat is the vortex for communication, oftentimes healing is as simple as speaking with someone you have not talked to for a long time. Begin a correspondence with the person you have failed to communicate with. If you feel they won't understand what you're saying, you could either be underestimating them or accurate in your assessment. In the latter case, it is better to handle your situation from within. During your daily meditation, open your heart and send that person compassion and watch your relationship grow deeper. And because communication is a two-way street, work on your listening skills, too.

Diarrhea

Diarrhea is usually an end result of too much worry. If you are brave enough to look beyond traditional thought, you will notice that this rarely occurs solely based on the foods you eat. There will be an emotional element involved either before, during, or after the meal you think caused it. Or, you may have developed intolerance for a particular type of food or ingredient based upon an emotional connection to an event that happened years ago! Either way, it is a symptom, not a cause. Recognize that you created the diarrhea and that you can un-create it—sometimes immediately.

Sometimes your body needs to detoxify—and fast. Though it may be unpleasant for just a little while, by knowing it is part of your own healing process, suffering can be diminished.

Skin Conditions

Adolescents' problematic skin is often blamed on the concept called puberty. Again, this may be true, but to accept puberty as the cause means you believe little can be done to alleviate the symptoms. If you look into the details of puberty, you will see that emotional repression is often the reason for the skin disorder. By the time puberty arrives, a teenager may worry and be fearful about the future, and feel anxious about the emerging and powerful lure of sexuality. Unfortunately, adults often do not guide and support teenagers in understanding these emotional states so that they can fully feel them, and then release them.

What is commonly called eczema, psoriasis, or even dandruff is also due to the repression of grief. Topical medications may help you feel better, but a good cry will help even more!

A Runny Nose

Stop self-medicating already! Your body needs to detoxify, and will eliminate what it perceives as toxins on its own, if you give it chance. Taking medication only stops the inherent and highly important detoxification process. By using a medication you may feel better initially, but you are stifling not curing the root cause. Buy a box of tissues, not a box of medication.

Learning Disabilities or Physical Handicaps

Some souls choose to incarnate with (or have a propensity toward experiencing) what we perceive as a disability. It may be either a means to teach the parents a lesson or be related to karma, or both. Usually, disability brings with it a very obvious compensatory gift. Kids labeled with Asperger's Syndrome, for example, are wonderfully artistic. Many kids diagnosed with autism are brilliant; expression is hampered by conventional standards, yet it is abundant in the psychic realms.

> *"When my son was given the diagnosis of cerebral palsy, I never told him what the diagnosis was. I just told him that he had some weak muscles and we had to work on them. I also told him that this was a blessing because it gave him a head start in life. He learned at an early age that things don't come easy and you have to work hard, but with that, a lot of positive things will happen. You value what you have and you feel you deserve it. He worked hard. Now, no one can tell that he has any muscular difficulty. He has learned how to compensate. It always amazes me that he is not even aware that at certain things he doesn't realize how hard he has to work. He thinks it is that way for everyone. That is his reality! He rides a bike and a scooter. And most importantly, he is a risk taker more than my other two children. I guess he knows it is okay to fall down. You just need to get back up and work harder."*
>
> —*ANONYMOUS CLIENT*

My client understood that labels disable, and labels that are thrown about have a tendency to disempower the individuals who are being labeled. By recognizing her child's strengths and seeing him as perfect and whole, she was able to instill in him high-quality values and self-confidence.

Some learning disabilities that are less severe can be created during childhood as an unconscious reaction to what is being perceived.

> *In second grade I couldn't pronounce the sound represented by "th" very well. I was put into a class with other learning disabled children, though we weren't called that. I don't remember if we were called anything in particular, but we definitely weren't called smart. I perceived that everyone thought something was very wrong with me.*

This type of labeling will have an effect on your expression and communication, of course. If a child feels they are being judged or labeled as stupid each time they speak, why would that youngster continue to speak? Why would they want to bring up further feelings of inadequacy?

Gas and Poor Digestion

This is usually the end result of eating too quickly and/or worrying while eating. Yes, it's that simple. The body's cells change instantly depending on your thoughts, and worry reduces the enzymes' ability to utilize the nutrition and energy from the foods being eaten. Obviously, it is very important to slow down and eat mindfully.

Sexual Dysfunction and Sexually Transmitted Diseases (STD)

Beyond obvious physical damage, sexual dysfunction is usually associated with learned and unnatural guilt and shame around innate and very natural thoughts and sensations. Shame and guilt actually block the natural and vibrant energy in the hips and genital regions and lead to problems. As shame and guilt increase, the body's immune response weakens. This increases the likelihood of contracting a sexually transmitted disease.

Testosterone and estrogen levels rise and fall with life's challenges and activities. If you're extremely passive, hate the work you're doing, or just don't feel like you're accomplishing anything on your mission, sexual performance can be affected. Stop looking at the disease and start looking at your life!

High Blood Pressure

If your muscles have tightened due to emotional toxicity such as anger, there is a good chance that they are either directly or indirectly constricting an artery or vein. This will obviously lead to internal arterial and/or venous pressure, making the heart work harder, and may lead to a diagnosis of high blood pressure.

Fortunately, there are effective medications for high blood pressure, but do you want to rely on those for the rest of your life? The only thing that will begin to reverse it naturally, without side effects and the best chance of permanent health, is to look deeply at and then purge the emotions that are causing it in the first place. In most cases, it is repressed anger. Even if you feel you don't have any issues, your body is saying otherwise. Most likely you were never given space or permission to feel your anger and had to hold it in. Even a tiny bit of anger can have an enormous effect on your body, so now imagine what months or decades of anger can do! You don't have to imagine, just look at your blood pressure monitor.

With her doctor's approval, a recent client weaned herself off her blood pressure medication while working with me. Her doctor didn't fully get what we were doing, but the results spoke for themselves! We identified the childhood scenarios that triggered anger and resentment. We then reprocessed the events that led her down that often gloomy, dead-end street. I taught her how to be proactive rather than reactive—a conscious creator as opposed to a victim of circumstance. That, combined with regular energy medicine sessions, did the job.

Anger, which is only one letter short of danger, will manifest in other forms as well. At the extreme, the condition commonly called cancer is often a result of stagnant energy from intense and prolonged repression of anger.

Diet is a factor in high blood pressure. Smoking, too, as it constricts blood flow. But you don't have to feel victimized by forces that cause you to smoke or eat junk food. Ask what it is that you are not willing to face that makes you seek to fill a perceived inner void with things that you know are bad for you. Identify *why* you are eating poorly, *why* you smoke, or *why* you need coffee every morning and after eating. Are you feeling sad, lonely, scared, anxious, or vengeful? What's the story behind your story?

If you are eating poorly or smoking, take a look at your self-esteem. Assuredly it has been compromised; why else would you ingest or breathe something that you know is harmful? If you need coffee in the morning, you are not getting enough quality sleep, and if you need it after a meal, you are either eating too much and/or eating foods that require too much energy to digest. Underneath it all is unprocessed anger that is dying to be released. More accurately, *you're* dying faster because you haven't yet released *it*. Your heart already works all day and night; don't make it work harder!

Mental Disorders

Because the mind and body are connected, and what happens in the former always manifests in the latter, what we call mental disorders often aren't mental disorders at all; they're the end results of emotional blockages. These blockages usually occur when someone is not given permission to feel their feelings.

The seemingly macho man who is living in fear from his abusive childhood never feels safe enough to be vulnerable and can even develop multiple personalities (besides Macho Man) to compensate. The child labeled with ADD is given medication to keep him calm, but no one seems to know why he's hyperactive, and some adults never even ask the question. The reality may be that he's just not interested in what this world is teaching him. These oft-gifted and highly misunderstood children already know much of what's being taught and seek challenges elsewhere. The fact that children labeled with ADD can focus on anything at all should tell you this label is false. That the youngster may not want to pay attention in school but can focus on a video game for hours should tell you it's the subject matter, not the child that needs to be addressed.

The ultra-likable woman who never gets upset, is diagnosed with depression, and people scratch their heads wondering how someone so sweet can end up with something so horrible. In many cases, doctors will analyze the brain and find levels of certain chemicals or neurotransmitters off from the proposed ideal. They may say that her depression is due to a low level of X, and then will recommend taking artificial X to get her back to normal; however, this does not work in the long term. This artificially induced version of normal may be better than being depressed temporarily, but it cannot heal her deep emotional wounds. She must be given space to feel her feelings and move the stagnant energy through emotional release work and/or see a practitioner who can move it with/for her with energy medicine.

Fears and Phobias

Without knowing where fear comes from, it is really tough to overcome it. I know someone who had a fear of doors. No one could figure out why or what to do about it, but she was determined to find out. Then one day she was given a vision. She "saw" a prior existence in which she was flattened by a falling door! Miraculously, so it would seem, after this vision her fear was gone. Sometimes, all it takes is an awareness of *why* and things begin to shift! Other times we have to allow ourselves to experience the fear in order to get over it. For example, people who have a fear of spiders can be helped by a professional who will coach them through an experience of having spiders walk on them, allowing them to overcome the phobia.

Insomnia

One of the most commonly misunderstood, and therefore misdiagnosed, maladies is sleeping difficulties. Uncountable numbers of insomniacs treat the symptoms with medications; however, few people feel more rested in the morning than they did before taking them. Why? Because the cause is not addressed: nighttime difficulties are developed during the daytime.

> *Leave your past behind, but never leave your behind in the past.*
> —AUDREY FUNG, DOCTOR OF OPTOMETRY

We are bombarded with advertising no matter where we go. Conversations begin and end with little actually said. Deadline stress tightens our physiology. And we worry about what to do, how to be, what others think, and where we're heading. Pressure builds up from so many sources, and we've no safe place to vent. The mind rambles on with projected scenarios or mistaken opportunities, and we expect it all to magically stop the moment we get horizontal after Letterman. This constant and oftentimes useless mind chatter can't just shut down the moment you lay down to rest; there is a buildup of energy that has to be released. You will sleep a thousand times better in quality, and you will be able to fall asleep instantly, when you give yourself a safe place to vent during the morning, afternoon, or early evening. Whether that's at the gym, on the dance floor or tennis court, or by journaling is irrelevant. Something must be done to quiet the mind and release the built-up energy.

"Anxiety"

Anxiety is highly misunderstood and, therefore, not permanently reversible in the typical healthcare paradigm. The condition usually described as anxiety is really a misunderstanding of time. While most grief is about regret from the past circling throughout the mind to no end, anxiety is an end result of fears of an as-yet-to-be-defined concept called the future. It's difficult to be anxious for more than a few moments when living in the now. If you are overly concerned with trying to control the future, it will take its toll on your physiology. Trying to control what can't be controlled is like standing before a tornado and pointing in another direction hoping it will grow eyes and consciousness to understand finger pointing and turn away. I may be wrong, but you just aren't that powerful yet, so why are you even trying? If you answered, "Because of my Ego," you're very right!

Hopelessness

Hopelessness is an end result of not trusting in the process. It is Ego at play. Even the moments seemingly encumbered with despair are surrounded with support; however, it's really difficult to feel that support when despondent. Yet even these moments in the grand scheme are totally perfect. Many people who have hit the highest points in life did so only after hitting rock bottom. Embrace the roller coaster. Hopelessness can be a chance to see the beauty of the challenges.

Spirit runs through you. Sometimes it is more noticeable than others. In moments of hopelessness, you're blocking the flow of energy within and from you, whereas, when in extreme joy, bliss takes over and hopelessness has little chance of survival.

Hopelessness is eradicated when you are doing and being that which brings you bliss. Likewise, bliss infuses you when you are doing whatever it is that you love most. This demonstration of passion within you is Spirit in motion.

If we all listened to spirit, imagine what we might become.
—PETRINA FISCHER WELLS, M.F.T., FOUNDER,
ADD INSTITUTE AND TREATMENT CENTER

For me, writing is a blissful demonstration of Spirit moving through me. For you it may be singing or cooking an exquisite meal. When you are doing that which you are "meant to do," time is irrelevant—meals go uneaten, calls go unreturned, the need for sleep is reduced, and there are even fewer visits to the bathroom! And, there is no room for hopelessness in bliss.

There are a thousand thoughts lying within a man that he
does not know till he takes up a pen to write.
—WILLIAM MAKEPEACE THACKERAY, AUTHOR

Does Worrying Affect Your Body?

Don't sweat the petty things, and don't pet the sweaty things.
—UNKNOWN WRITER

When you persist in harboring lower-vibration thoughts (complaints, blame, and so on), you only draw forth more situations about which to complain and blame. This weakens the immune system. If you continue, you may reduce your immune system's efficiency to such a low point it can't even fight off the common cold any longer.

Some people spend their whole lives worrying about money, health, or even the littlest of things. There are those people who worry about all they've done, all they are doing, and all that they might one day do. Then there are those people who worry about money, health, or even the littlest things *in other people* in addition to worrying about money, health, or even the littlest things *in themselves*!

NOTE: *Worry is the activity of a mind that is disconnected from Source.*

When you worry about things you can't change, you are creating useless, disintegrative energy, or energy that destroys. Why concern yourself with things that are totally out of your control? Does it make any sense to worry about the outcome of the Lakers game? They're probably going to win anyway. (As a Knicks fan, the NBA has been a sore subject for me the last few years.) Does it make any sense to worry about people you don't even know? Why do we watch chat shows on television or read gossip magazines? How does it affect your life knowing what Brad Pitt is doing? Are you going to invite him to your home for Thanksgiving? When worried about a loved one, for example, we can let our mind wonder about potential worst-case scenarios or just pick up the phone and know within seconds that our family members are alright.

NOTE: *Worry is a deconstructive thought process that requests the Universe provide you exactly what you don't really want.*

If you've been worrying for so long that it's become a way of life, how do you release it? You do so by intently looking at what you are worrying about. The more you look at it, the more it will disappear.

> *We have gotten into the habit of spending money we haven't earned,*
> *to buy things we don't need, to impress people that we don't like.*
> *So get rid of that habit.*
> —DR. DEEPAK CHOPRA, SPIRITUAL TEACHER AND AUTHOR

Let's say, you are worried about money. You constantly worry that you do not have enough and as a result, you will be so disheartened and respond so inadequately that you will never have enough! You will be borrowing from friends and family (or the guy in the trench coat), using credit cards, looking to see what junk you can sell, attempting to cut costs ("Who needs toilet paper, anyway?"), all while sending out the energy that not only created this but is also keeping it in place. Now, look at the subject of this worry and ask yourself, "What is the worst thing that can happen?" And then ask yourself, "And then what?" Answer honestly with the first thing that comes to mind. And then ask "And then what?" once again! If you're letting the answer come from your heart and not your Ego, the worry will break down right in front of you. Your heart will guide you to a solution if you let it.

If you are worrying about not having enough food to eat, note there is more food being wasted every day in America than is eaten on a given day in many other countries. Here in the United States, you have to work really hard to starve. In fact, many "Freegans" eat for free, even if they can afford to pay for food, by eating the discarded food from restaurants and grocery stores! If you are worried about employment, you can get a job—any job. Release pride and face reality; you can even receive food stamps until you get a job if necessary. There are always alternatives, only our pride stops us from seeing them. I was on food stamps a few years ago until I made a change. In some parts of the world, there are people who live over a year on what you make in a week. All things are relative, and it is important to see this to remind yourself of how good you have it.

> *Death is a horizon, and a horizon is but a limit to our sight.*
> —*PRESIDENT ABRAHAM LINCOLN*

What else could one worry about? Well, what made you pick up this book? Your health, of course. What is the worst that can happen in matters of your health? Most fear being in lots of pain and dying. That's not real comforting, is it? But what if death did not exist? That is to say, what if death, as we have believed it to be, were a myth? Would that knowledge be enough to release all your worry?

> *There are no unnatural or supernatural phenomena,*
> *only very large gaps in our knowledge.*
> —*EDGAR MITCHELL, ASTRONAUT*

Of course "death" exists, but I would suggest, based on my own channeled messages and New Age philosophy, that it is probably nothing like what our more popular theologies have made it out to be, and that is where and why our worries began. The life of your soul is peaceful and eternal, but we've been conditioned to believe it is filled with pain, judgment, and more pain. This is the work of fear-filled oppressors—not that of a loving, compassionate God.

NOTE: *The swami pointed out: When a baby is born and the soul enters the outer physical realm, the baby cries, yet the family rejoices. When an old man is about to pass and his soul is about to leave the realm of the physical, the family cries, yet the old man is peaceful.*

You don't need to take my word for this. There are numerous believable accounts of reincarnation. One book, *Many Lives, Many Masters* by Dr. Brian Weiss, is the true story of how a Western-trained and highly prominent psychiatrist and the head of his department in a major hospital put his reputation on the line by publicly sharing his experiences with a client who, when under hypnosis, could talk about her past lifetimes. He then tells how that information was used in her therapy sessions to alleviate her symptoms in the present. For me, the most interesting thing in this book is the author's consistent disbelief until the evidence was so strong that he had to give in to this being real, despite it being fully against everything he'd ever known. How many of you can relate to that?

Maybe this world is another planet's Hell.
—ALDOUS HUXLEY, NOVELIST

For more evidence that death itself is not to be feared, you could also spend some time with Dannion Brinkley. He's been hit by lightning twice and has survived three near-death-experiences (NDE), where he was on the other side and then came back to tell his tale. Also, famous mediums like James Van Praagh communicate quite effectively with those who have left the body. How would he be able to share all the things he hears if there was no life after death? It is only our quite common fear-based theologies that do not let us look at the concept of death as anything other than choices between existent versions that include myths of Heaven and Hell. Heaven is all things that are beautiful right here and right now, and Hell is anything but. If you are living your gift of life wastefully, you are creating your own Hell. If you are living in fear of an afterlife in Hell, you are not living, but rather are already creating it and dying there.

I've listed some of the most common pains, illnesses, and seemingly negative situations above. While your particular condition may not have been listed, the commonalities among ailments should be apparent. For further information, feel free to use the tools in upcoming chapters. If that still isn't enough, please attend a workshop or book a private session, even by phone, for your individualized needs.

CHAPTER 3

Tools to Raise Awareness

Obviously, awareness of the underlying causes of pains and illness is paramount. In fact, it's the first step in The Five Steps to Health, which I will explain shortly. So how does one raise this awareness?

1. The Mind-Body Worksheet

If you are experiencing any discomfort in this moment, you can assist your process of seeing it with new eyes by doing the mind-body worksheet. This will assist in changing your perspective so that you can begin to change a physical symptom. Even the physical is not as dense as we once believed. We're all made of energy that can be transformed at the tiniest levels of existence. This transformation of thought immediately catalyzes transformation on the physical level.

Draw a line straight across the top of a page. On top of it, write out ONE pain you are currently experiencing.

EXAMPLE: Shoulder pain

Draw a second line underneath it. On top of that line, write down what aggravates this pain.

EXAMPLE: It hurts when I carry a heavy bag

Draw a third line underneath these two. Answer, "What does this activity mean to me?"

EXAMPLE: It feels like I have the weight of the whole world on my shoulders

In this example, you have determined what is causing your shoulder pain with no help needed from an outside source. In just a few moments, you now have information to release your pain, whereas moments before you drew blanks. Using this example, check to see if you really have the weight of the whole world on your shoulders—a colloquialism for carrying the burden of too much responsibility—or if you just think you do. Odds are pretty high that you just think you do. This does not diminish the pain or the situation you are experiencing at all; but it helps in realizing how you've hurt yourself by carrying this self-created responsibility. Knowing that you created this pain shows that you can get rid of it, too!

2. The Stress Test

A common link among most pains or illness is stress, or shall we say, *perceived* stress. Stress can mean a lot of things to a lot of different people, but we will attempt to simplify the process here. Check off which of the following potential stressors you feel are causing you stress, and write down any additional unnamed stressors where it says, "Other." Afterward, there will be a rating scale and a full, detailed, thought-provoking explanation of the category you fit into, and more importantly, information and suggestions on what you can do to alleviate stress entirely.

☐ Work   ☐ Family
☐ Relationships   ☐ Money
☐ Car   ☐ Deadlines
☐ Pressure   ☐ Noise
☐ Toxins, environmental and other   ☐ Pollution
☐ Being cut off on the highway   ☐ Being bumped into on the street
☐ Emotional trauma   ☐ Injuries
☐ Landlords   ☐ Government
☐ Religion   ☐ This book
☐ Other:_____

Now count the number of check marks you've made and rate yourself according to the following profiles:

If you checked off 13 or more, you are a "MIS" personality.

If you checked off 9–12, you are an "IN" personality.

If you checked off 5–8, you are a "FORM" personality,

If you checked off 1–4, you are an "ED" personality...

Now add up all the "types" of personalities and . . .

Oops, looks like you've been… **MIS−IN−FORM− ED!**

Gotcha!

Not a single one of these items is a cause of stress! It is only your perception of them that makes them appear stress inducing. If you think that your family causes you stress, you are mistaken—it is your reaction to your family that does it. If you feel your relationship is causing your stress, you have been misguided—it is your perspective on it that does. If you think your job causes you stress, you have been misled—it is your reaction to it where the problem lies.

If it was only your job, for example, EVERYONE who has that same type of job would be equally stressed. Obviously, this is not the case. There are stressed-out lawyers and there are lawyers who look at the exact same situation and see it as a challenge or a labor of love. The trick is seeing with a new perspective—looking at it with new eyes and asking yourself, "How can I be with X, and feel different about it?" "Can I see my deadline as a challenge instead of a burden?" "Can I see my partner as caring and not overbearing?" "Can I see my family as those who love me in their own way, and not those who annoy me?" Do this on your own or work with an intuitive practitioner or a trusted friend who will guide you to your own answers and elicit more questions.

NOTE: *It is time to forgive where you once held anger. It is time for wisdom where you once only had knowledge. It is time to accept where once you were judgmental. It is time to love where you once held fear.*

3. Listening to Your Body

To the mind that is still,
the whole universe surrenders.
—*LAO-TZU, PHILOSOPHER*

As a medical intuitive, I have come to realize that our bodies are always telling us what is going on, but we are too busy in our thoughts to hear it. Begin by bringing attention to the area of discomfort. Breathe deeply and be open. Let go of any thoughts about the pain itself; release judgments, *should haves, shouldn't haves,* and so on, and lovingly ask, "What message do you have for me?" Then stay with the silence without any judgments and listen closely for the answer. The message or the method of its transmission may not be what you expect. Stay open. You may get a feeling, a memory, a picture, or even an idea. You may hear a song in the background or taste something that's not even in your mouth. Just by staying open, you too, can become your own medical intuitive!

50

I asked Andrea to do this about her ankle sprain. She replied "I've just always had weak ankles, and walking in four-inch heels for work doesn't help."

I reminded her that other women who do the same job don't always have weak ankles. We needed to find out why she was having these problems while others didn't. I asked her to ask her own ankle what was going on. Andrea centered herself and after a few minutes got a message that this job was not her ultimate calling, and to stop treating it that way. When she dedicated more time to writing, even while wearing high heels to work, her ankle began to heal.

4. Meditation

The surest path to the soul is to clear the mind with regular meditation. Soul is the home of your truth and that of the collective unconscious. A quiet mind can enable you to more effectively monitor your thoughts. The mind-body connection promoted by regular meditation can be extremely beneficial in helping you to attain and maintain optimum health. A clear mind, even it's only for a few moments, will put you more in touch with your Truth. Truth lies within your heart and soul. The quality of being that you enjoy when you are in touch with your heart and soul (a unified state) is quite unlike that of working with the mind (a place of dualistic thinking). When you connect with your heart and soul, beliefs about what is true or what you've heard from friends or even some practitioners simply dissolve in the face of a clear "felt sense" of Absolute Truth that is quiet and unshakable. When you connect with your heart and soul, you listen and receive guidance; you don't do the guiding.

There is no shortage of excellent how-to manuals that offer instruction on how to meditate. In general, most meditation instructions suggest beginning a practice by connecting with your breath. So take a deep breath right now. Place your hands on your abdomen to feel the giving and receiving of air deep into your body. Concentrate on the out-breath. On the purely physical level, this will help calm you because deep breathing sends a signal to the body that you are relaxed, and the body will follow and relax as well. Focus on a mantra, your breath, or a particular sensation. If you notice yourself mentally drifting, do not beat yourself up for it and merely go back to where you were.

Most men pursue pleasure with such
breathless haste they hurry past it.
—*SOREN KIERKEGAARD, PHILOSOPHER*

Of course, we will want to get results immediately, and some of us will. If you do not, release the learned perfectionism and try again later. Or, see if this is symbolic of how you deal with other things in your life. Do you always have to succeed? Do you often look for the quicker but less efficient method? Do you give up too quickly? At least *try* to enjoy the process. By meditating each day, even for only 15 minutes, you will feel more relaxed, centered, and calm, and have greater access to your intuition—where all the awareness we could ever ask for resides!

> NOTE: *Perfectionism is an invitation to disappointment. Let this be an opportunity to experience self-compassion!*

Meditation will also enable you to hear beyond your personal space—what is going on "out there." You will be better attuned to the feelings of others and begin to see them as they really are. Awareness of both the joy and the pain of others increases, and you will be better able to lend a hand as needed—as well as know what type of a hand to give. Here are some different meditations to try, some alone, some in groups:

GROUP BODY LISTENING: Sit with your knees touching those of another person. Spend a few moments in silence together. Then ask out loud, repeatedly if need be, "What is causing my _____?" (Fill in the blank with your pain or illness.) If the other individual is centered, she will receive messages she can share with you. Then, reverse the process. The revelations that come through can be remarkable. Make it fun. With group body listening, you will be amazed at what others can tell you, and what you will tell them! You may hear what you've always needed to hear, or share what someone else has needed to hear. That's why we have each other!

MUSIC: There are many types of music that can assist your meditation practice; some persons are moved by classical, others by ambient or New Age. Music can be a powerful tool in our physical, mental, emotional, and spiritual healing process. Recorded music carries the energy of the performer with it. If listened to with openness, the musician's intent can be transferred to the listener.

> *Music is a higher revelation than philosophy.*
> —*LUDWIG VAN BEETHOVEN, COMPOSER*

When used with conscious intention, the healing effects of music can be far and wide. See how you feel when listening to a particular piece of music versus another. Are you invigorated or angered? Strengthened or weakened? Is your mind clear or wandering? Music can bring you to a more relaxed state to increase your awareness of what is really going on in your body just by setting that as intention before you begin listening.

Many people chant to bring themselves to ecstasy, oftentimes in a group environment. Besides any religious connection, there is a scientific reason for this. Energy, like water, seeks its own level when you're open to that being so. When you enter a room of chanters, often just by being there you, too, will have a higher vibration. Of course, if you want to judge, make fun, or pick out who has the worst voice, you can do that, too. But doing so is not helpful in raising your vibration.

> *Music for me is proof of the existence of God*
> —*KURT VONNEGUT, AUTHOR*

Some people use chanting to draw the spirit world to them. They "call in" the directions or various spirit guides. While it certainly isn't a bad thing for the "(w)hol(l)y spirit" to visit, you can do something that is even more beneficial. Anything you do to raise your vibration, which is often easier in a room filled with like-minded people, brings you that much closer to the spirit world. By the laws of quantum physics, you will feel lighter and eventually mesh with Spirit in its realm, as well as be able to hear what's going on within!

NOTE: *See* www.BarryGoldstein.com *for excellent ambient music!*

PHYSICAL EXERCISE: Whether you use your body to calm the mind, or calm the mind to relax the body is irrelevant; both are important to wellbeing. Among the many methods for clearing the mind are exercise, and none that I know are more powerful than yoga. One of the reasons why yoga is so powerful is that when you perform most *asanas*, or yogic postures, you concentrate on keeping your balance and breathing. You can't worry about paying your rent or you'll fall. In a way, it is forced mind relaxation! In general, the more calming and focusing the activity, the more relaxed the mind will become, making it easier to hear answers to your questions.

When working with any of the above, the most important thing you can do is to set a specific intention beforehand. Music can be relaxing or invigorating. Meditation can be used to increase awareness or to become one with Spirit. Likewise, if you've already got a clear vision of the underlying cause of your pain or illness but haven't been able to purge it, you can set an intention before your next meditation to get the answer to the question of "Why not? What next step should I take that I am not seeing?"

CHAPTER 4

The Five Steps to Health

Step 1: Awareness

We already know that awareness is absolutely crucial to healing and more importantly, preventing, pain and illness. If we were aware that anger, for example, can cause serious chronic pain or worse, we would do anything to avoid being angry, right? So how do we avoid becoming angry? We don't!

Life isn't about not getting angry. Until you're enlightened, you will get angry. Avoiding it is pretty tough, but by practicing proactive/conscious behavior as opposed to reactive/unconscious behavior, it can certainly be minimized. To maintain health and prevent illness, it is imperative to recognize the anger as soon as possible and either release it physically in a safe environment or reprocess the situation. The former can even be done by beating a pillow with a plastic bat. The energy must be moved somehow; the worst thing you can do is to repress it.

All emotions are based on thoughts and perceptions. Change those and you minimize reactions. Take for example the understanding in some societies that death is a release from suffering. Those people, who we think would typically mourn, don't suffer with nearly the same levels of grief as we do in the West. Though they may miss the person, incidences of ailments related to grief repression such as asthma or obesity in those cultures are few and far between. However it's a tricky distinction between thinking yourself out of feeling a certain way and truly not feeling that way. Ego will want you to think you're above grieving, when in reality you're not 100 percent sure that death is a release. The emotion and the corresponding energy that's created ends up stagnating in your body—that's not what we're looking for here. It takes an honest introspection that may be extremely difficult for even an advanced practitioner of the healing arts. We highly recommend an intuitive and compassionate practitioner to guide you.

Let us not confuse healthy emotions with unhealthy emotions. There's nothing wrong with grieving for a deceased loved one. In fact, it's healthy to do so. The problems come when we begin to feel the sadness and either stifle it completely or become so attached to it that, in time, we identify with it. Perhaps it's a way of hooking the attention of others, or perhaps you feel good in your misery.

The occasional release of grief allows for its equal and opposite reaction: an enhanced ability to express joy. They're two sides of the same coin. All of our natural emotions are expressions of a side of humanity that we are told to suppress; yet they make us who we are. We need to honor them, not push them away. Fear, love, anger, grief, and envy are natural states; however, when they're repressed, it may lead you to experience these and other symptoms:

- Repressed fear can lead to external blame, anxiety, panic, and neurological conditions (for example, what is called tremors/Parkinson's), and more.
- Repressed love leads to neediness, obsession, unbalanced relationships, heart and circulation problems, and more.
- Repressed anger becomes muscle tightness, hatred, physical aches and pains, tumors, rage, violence, and more.
- Repressed grief leads to skin, sinus, breathing, and elimination problems; pancreatic dysfunction; apathy; depression; and more.
- Repressed envy leads to jealousy, theft, insecurity, and more.
- Repressed worry can lead to victim consciousness, *spleen* problems, digestive disorders, poor appetite, bloating, weakness in the limbs, and more.

So let us summarize what can be very confusing here. Until you are really good at staying in the present, and until you fully understand how things work and can truly be proactive rather than reactive, it's best to feel the emotions and move the associated energy or have it moved with or for you. When you get to live in higher vibrations, you can better integrate the experiences that used to bring you down and let them pass right through you.

When emotions are repressed, it creates an energetic weakness, meaning that energy does not flow but rather is blocked. People with energetic blockages are now more susceptible to physical injury than others. Indeed, uncountable numbers of people have played tennis or worked a keyboard, and have experienced pain. And there are uncountable others who did the exact same motions with the exact same amount of exertion who were not diagnosed with tennis elbow or carpal tunnel syndrome. If it was only the physical force that injured people, everyone who experienced these movements would be hurt in the same way. That is obviously not the case. So, does tennis cause tennis elbow? Does working at a computer cause carpal tunnel syndrome? Does lifting something heavy always cause back pain? What do *you* think?

Awareness, although highly atypical, is a state of mind that consistently and eventually quite naturally involves keen perception of all possible perspectives around and within any persons or situation. Awareness means mindfulness of who and what is around us, how they or it are affecting us, and how we are affecting them.

Step 2: Acceptance

Whatever the present moment contains, accept it as if you had chosen it.
Accept—then act. Always work with it, not against it.
Make the present your friend and ally, not your opponent.
This will miraculously transform your whole life.
—ECKHART TOLLE, AUTHOR

Because thoughts are creative, complaining about what *shouldn't be* is further re-creating *what already is*. The creative forces of the Universe that are put into motion by your thoughts do not differentiate between *should be*'s and *shouldn't be*'s; they simply re-create the subject matter of the sentence. Your thoughts—and, therefore, your energy toward the subject of what you feel *shouldn't be*—actually re-creates what you feel shouldn't be! I know that concept sounds dumb, but when you talk to the Creator you can tell Her to do it differently next time; for now we need to play by Her rules!

Resistance is futile.
—THE BORG

Try thinking or saying "I am healthy," or if that seems too unrealistic right now, try "All things lead to being healthy," as opposed to saying, "There *shouldn't be* pain." You will then be giving energy toward creating health as opposed to creating energy leading to pain. It is more positive to say, "There *can be* peace" than "there *shouldn't be* war" because you are giving energy to peace. Think about all the aspects of you that are healthy:

> *She feels her leg muscles flex and relax when she walks up the stairs. She listens to her tireless heart beating rhythmically in the dance of life. He can touch her skin; it's soft and flexible like her wide open heart. She moves with ease known only by water. Her body is a flowing spiral of unbreakable energy; he can bend and twist and run, and she embraces the all. They can see their breath on a chilly winter morning. They can hear the laughter of a baby who is just starting to walk.*

Those who live in the land of *should be* and *shouldn't be* tend to resist what is, and often complain a lot. And anyone who consistently complains about their ill health takes forever to heal because they are re-feeding the causative energy! Resistance is the exact opposite of acceptance. Yet, many of these same people will also not tell others of upcoming good news in fear of jinxing it!

For some people, the word *acknowledgment* is a better description of this concept. Either way, acceptance doesn't mean giving up on changing something, nor does it mean to say, "Hooray, I have herpes!" In fact it's quite the opposite. When you accept what is, as it is, when it is, you are creating room for something new. Lack of acceptance of what is, or resistance, re-creates what it is that you don't like. An obvious example of this is that fighting for peace through modes of violence only propagates the fighting. And even if it seems to diminish it temporarily—because the energy is burying rather than healing, it will return with even more vengeance.

Step 3: Opportunity

Once you are fully aware of what caused your pain or illness and have accepted it, you will have an opportunity to look into an emotional aspect of yourself in need of healing. We already know that complaining about a thing you don't really want will just keep it in place; continued complaining manifests into chronic pain or more serious illness.

If your pain is a result of repressed anger, look at it as an opportunity to investigate that anger and understand why it is there, and then figure out what to do about it. Ask yourself, "How can I be with this anger in a way that is more *creative* than *destructive* to my health and to my life?" This simple step can heal old relationships and clear unfinished business, which will alleviate your symptoms with no negative side effects!

Seeing pain or illness as an opportunity and not a burden is a key to spiritual growth and improving physical health. Two persons might view the same task from different perspectives: one will see it as a challenge and, therefore, love it; and the other will be miserable. Guess which one will have better health! When you can view things—even an illness—as an opportunity, that alone can decrease some of your symptoms. Now you are more able to feel the ever-present healing love that always is there.

"My shoulder hurts when I raise my arm, so I cannot do yoga this week."
Yeah, and … ?

While not being able to do something you consider beneficial may initially feel like a burden, you can practice acceptance by taking this opportunity to try something else. Maybe it's time to take a walk in a park and feel the fresh air invigorate you as much as a hatha yoga class might. Maybe you can jog around the block a few times, or even start a project that gives your shoulder a rest. See things as an opportunity and not a burden, and watch what happens. When you have really mastered seeing things as an opportunity, the next step is to see everything and everyone as a gift. For all things and people truly are a gift; we did nothing to deserve anything, much less life itself.

Step 4: Gratitude

Feeling grateful or appreciative of someone or something in your life
actually attracts more of the things that you appreciate and value into your life.
—*DR. CHRISTIANE NORTHROP, AUTHOR*

Complaining about what you do not have creates distance between you and your perceived missing piece. Conversely, simply being thankful for those things we already have has the effect of attracting more and better-quality things to us! It could be a lot worse. If you can read this book, be thankful you are among those who can read. If you can afford to buy nice clothing, be thankful that you have a job that probably makes you more money in a day than most of the world's population earns in a year. There is always something to be thankful for.

She witnesses her own smile while watching herself in the mirror as she laughs with joy from watching herself in the mirror! She touches the fur of her cat as he purrs with delight. She hears the words of Rumi from her lover's lips, and tastes their love in the air between them. She feels her connection to the divine and all that is, and smells the flowers outside her door—even after they are long gone—with just a memory of their scent.

You can be thankful for your car, your fingers, water, the sun, or even something that initially seems horrible such as high blood pressure or even cancer. How many people have taken their lives for granted until they're threatened with a serious condition? Afterward, many of these people will claim to feel a rebirthing. There is now a new opportunity to do things differently; they received and answered their wake-up call!

To speak gratitude is courteous and pleasant.
To enact gratitude is generous and noble,
but to live gratitude is to touch Heaven.
—*JOHANNES A. GAERTNER, CONSULTANT*

A more tangible aspect of the gratitude phase is called *listing*. Even if you are mad at someone, list three things every day, even if they are the same three things repeated each day, that were positive about that person or your experience with that person. Take time to meditate on these positive aspects. This is one method of feeling and expressing gratitude, thus reinforcing those positive, healing energies, as opposed to repeating the creation of the negative energy pattern that got you in pain to begin with!

> *Here is my wish for you and every other child, woman, and man on the face*
> *of the earth: Spend one week saying only kind, caring things to yourself.*
> *Say thank you at least ten times an hour, direct five toward yourself and*
> *five to the world at large. Compliment yourself (and others) each time an*
> *effort is made. Notice all the wonderful qualities and characteristics about*
> *yourself and those around you. One week. You will never go back. And your*
> *whole life will be a glorious meditation.*
>
> —*CHERI HUBER, AUTHOR*

Many of us are taught by organized religions to believe that God would be more inclined to grant us our wishes *if* we express gratitude. I'm sorry to burst your egocentric bubble, but this is an example of human projection upon the Creator. In actuality, as we increase the loving feelings generated by the inward or outward expression of gratitude, our vibration increases. And that calls forth more of the positive! Gratitude creates space and leads to a considerably easier time with the next step—the ultimate of healers—forgiveness.

Step 5: Forgiveness

> *Life is for–giving, not for–getting.*
> —*NEALE DONALD WALSH, AUTHOR*

Steps 1 through 4 lead to forgiveness, one of the most powerful healing forces in the universe! This concept brings up a lot of questions about blame, vengeance, and justice. How can we forgive even the most grievous of crimes? How can we forgive when all we've been taught about any wrongdoing is to seek justice, or even vengeance? It begins by altering the parameters around the definition of forgiveness itself!

> *Living in the old paradigm of love, he was angry for not getting what he was*
> *taught he should be getting from his girlfriend. He was blinded by love's allure; he*
> *could not feel his own pain when in her presence. He built up a lot of anger toward*

her for something she had not only little idea about, but didn't have the desire to see. He thought he had to forgive her, but how could he forgive someone who had no idea of how her actions were affecting him? Later, he realized he had to forgive himself.

Take steps to become aware of why someone did something to you that you perceive as harmful, and fully understand that no one does anything they think is wrong. All actions are justified, or they are left undone. As difficult as this is to believe, it has to be true. You would not, ever, do what you feel is wrong. If you did something while thinking it was wrong, you would have to justify it to make it okay, thereby making it right, even if only temporarily. Your perpetrator was taught their reality. He had to have justified his actions based on what he'd been taught. Another possibility is that his Ego self got too powerful and began to override his heart. For you to heal it is imperative to see the situation from beyond your filtered, hurt point of view.

Forgiveness is the correction of perception.
—*A COURSE IN MIRACLES*

You don't forgive by letting someone off the hook; that does nothing but repress your emotions further. You forgive by altering the definition of forgiveness, from "letting someone off the hook" to "canceling their effects on you." You claim to yourself and the Universe that you have learned not to repress anger—that you have learned from this opportunity that no one is perfect and everyone makes mistakes.

If you want others to be happy, practice compassion.
If you want to be happy, practice compassion.
—*THE DALAI LAMA*

Utilize compassion here, for it is just another amazing tool in the healing of the self and the planet. By exhibiting compassion, forgiveness becomes easy! Besides, having compassion just feels good. With compassion comes the realization that mistakes are really not mistakes at all, but are opportunities to learn what types of behavior are best not repeated.

NOTE: *When I was unable to be diagnosed by ten different doctors for the same set of symptoms, I held anger towards them. This delayed and actually prevented healing until I realized they were doing their best, given their model of healing.*

You don't have to experience every wrongdoing, mistake, or resultant anger on your own. You can learn from the actions of others. You can decide to forgive, or cancel, the perception of an alleged perpetrator's mistakes because not forgiving is too painful to your own self. You forgive because you realize through your own awareness that an assumed perpetrator is really a gift (in the larger picture) in disguise. You forgive because you love yourself too much not to do so. You forgive by utilizing *the* most powerful force in the Universe—Love.

CHAPTER 5

Choosing Love

Maybe love is letting people be just who they need to be.
—*HOWARD JONES, SINGER/SONGWRITER*

Love is the glue of life. Love heals all because love IS all. When in doubt, always choose love. How? Before doing anything ask yourself, "Am I doing this from a state of love or from a state of fear?" By inquiring into this *before* reacting (literally, to act again) to any situation, you are assured of always doing the right thing (right being subjective—we mean while considering all of the variables leading to greater understanding, harmony, and health). Even if your initial reaction is out of Ego or fear, take a step back as soon as possible and view things through a larger perspective. Call upon the love of your Creator, spirit guides, family member, partner, family pet, or even the love of yourself for guidance.

> NOTE: *In the absence of love there is fear, and fear is a powerful, creative force. What you fear, you will eventually create. You now can love where you once held fear by making that conscious decision to be love in any moment.*

All too often, we slip out of our inherent state of love because we have been conditioned to do so. At that moment, anything is possible, so try to recognize that you are coming from fear and use the Five Steps to Health! You are now **aware** that you erred; you can **accept** that you did; you see the **opportunity** you have created; you can express **gratitude**; and you can **forgive** yourself, thereby setting the conditions for the re-creation of love in your mind, body, and soul.

If you fear making a presentation in front of a large group of people, you're not alone. But if you fill your mind and body with love, attendees are going to love you. Great actors and performers know that if they throw their whole selves into the performance, they'll be respected and appreciated. Have faith in who you are and what you are doing and others will, too.

As time goes on, the "down-time" between states of love will decrease. You may ride the emotional roller coaster for as long as you like, but why would you choose to do that? When looking through the eyes of unconditional love, all can be understood, all can be accepted, and all can be forgiven. *All can be healed.*

> *For every moment of truth, there's confusion in life.*
> *Love can be seen as the answer.*
> —*RONNIE JAMES DIO, SINGER, SONGWRITER*

When you monitor your thoughts more attentively and catch yourself before becoming engulfed in the conditioning from your past, you can make a new decision in each moment. Do this every hour if that's what it takes. When you catch yourself thinking of the negative, invite yourself to the next highest thought. Actually say, "I invite the next highest thought to mind" (but maybe not out loud on the subway). Clarity shortly follows—about everything!

> *We are not held back by the love we didn't receive in the past;*
> *but by the love we're not extending in the present.*
> —*UNKNOWN AUTHOR*

Love as you have been taught is conditional. True love is unconditional. Unconditional love allows each person to be whoever they choose to be. Conditional love binds. Unconditional love frees. Conditional love is why relationships do not work. Unconditional love is why they do. Conditional love is the norm in most younger-culture societies (what many call "civilized" cultures), as opposed to tribal, communal, or older cultures that don't hold back the natural flow of love. Conditional love is the more human and very typical expression we confuse as true love when there is often only intense "like." We learn about conditional love from those who raised us, stories in religious text, and even what we're told about Santa Claus—that he'll only give us presents if we are "good." Even jolly Saint Nick has an agenda!

> *Falling in love you remain a child;*
> *rising in love you mature.*
> —*OSHO*

The current understanding of falling in love is quite beautiful, and maybe even worth all the effort of attaining it, but having these perfect scenarios of total and permanent bliss with the perfect partner constantly in your mind could lead to disappointment. So practice love unconditionally and rise in love with everyone and everything and see how you feel.

Love's passion became unbridled from its inner, bottled up life, and overtook my mind, filling this body with warmth and light. Like when you were a child running toward no place in particular and laughing at what isn't even funny. Like when you sang at the top of your lungs without caring whether you're bothering anyone, or if you were even remotely in key! I got lost in my lover's eyes and melted into her. Feeling the walls morph around us and feeling every fear and every hurt and anguish we've ever had, never once did I take my gaze from hers.

CHAPTER 6

Why Choose Fear?

The workshop leader calmly lit the gauze-wrapped end of an aluminum rod and the flames rose, reaching 10 or more inches in height. He tilted his head back and placed the lit end into his mouth and closed his lips around the flames. He then opened his mouth and took out the rod, smiling, unscathed. "Now, you're going to do it!" he announced to a roomful of about 1,000 people. My reply: "Huh? We're all going to eat fire? Um, can I get the check, please?!" Most of the audience had a similar reaction.

The workshop leader explained how our fears hold us back from living a life we love. This training was a reminder that we can overcome fear that we normally experience with determination and perseverance. Granted, some fears are really necessary. If a car is coming at you at a really high speed, fear will most likely be the reaction and give you the strength to get out of the way in time. A good thing, for sure.

Fear is not healthy when we are reacting to a situation that isn't life-threatening as if it were life-threatening. When we let our fears win, we live a life of quiet desperation. Most of our fears are projections into a possible, though ultimately imaginary future. But our bodies react as if that situation was happening right then and there. Who hasn't had thoughts about an upcoming event and felt nervous, anxious, even scared; yet, those are all reactions that need not occur. Why? Because the causes are not real. In that moment, they're a projection, and odds are high that it's your rampaging mind that made you fearful.

If we continue to live in this illusory world, it will eventually catch up with us emotionally and physically. The body responds to fight-or-flight reactions to stress in numerous ways. We're instantly prepared to stay and deal with the situation or to flee. Blood pressure rises and adrenaline is pumped throughout the body, and that's a good thing. But logically speaking, if the fear is not dealt with at that time, stress becomes a way of life—even unconsciously—and over the long term this is actually quite detrimental to health.

One reaction to fear is body shaking, even if minimal. If the body shakes from a little bit of fear, what's going to happen when fear is omnipresent? What if—even unconsciously—someone remains trapped in the never-ending mind game of reacting to situations as burdens? What about those who continue to create unnecessary detrimental bodily reactions to often unreal situations? On the emotional level, anxiety becomes pervasive. And if the fear is both prolonged and intense over a lengthy period of time, lots of shaking is seen, a condition known as Parkinson's.

No one can live a life without obstacles; it's not part of the plan. What makes some people thrive and others merely survive is their reaction to these obstacles. We can choose to let anything become a burden or an opportunity. Either way, it is our choice.

The workshop leader acknowledged the real danger in eating fire and gave us a few tips. "Don't burn your mouth" was certainly helpful. He then gave us a few more useful instructions and said, "If I can do it, so can all of you." So when presented with a 10-inch flame as my obstacle, I and a thousand others agreed this was an opportunity! We used the flame as a metaphor for real-life situations; for example, when the boss threatened us to shape up or ship out, or when we found out we had an illness, or had a difficult family situation.

I got excited at the challenge and at the same time thought, "I'll do it, but I'm not gonna be first!" And after the first few people did it, I somehow summoned the courage to do it, too. I figured "If they can do it, so can I." (Note: DO NOT TRY THIS AT HOME—WE WERE TAUGHT HOW TO DO IT BY PROFESSIONALS!) Next thing I knew, a thousand people lined up to eat fire. One by one, cheering each other on, we lit the gauze, tipped back our heads and ate fire! And no one got burned.

So when life presents you with an unexpected curveball, you, too, can see it as an opportunity rather than a burden and tackle it. Directly face the fear when possible. And stop worrying about what could be—or worse—complaining about what is, and ask yourself if others have gone through something similar and survived. Then do as we did: say to yourself, "If they can do it, so can I!"

CHAPTER 7

Healing Deeper Layers of Pain

"Health is a means, not an end.
Good health allows us to do the work we're meant to do.
Conversely, doing the work we're meant to do gives us good health."
—ANNEMARIE COLBIN, PH.D, AUTHOR

The Five Steps to Health are great for maintaining health and preventing pain and illness from manifesting in your life and body. They can be used quite effectively for understanding and reversing what might be considered minor pains and illness. But what can you do if, through awareness, you realize that what you're dealing with has several layers of emotional trauma? What if you've spent a good deal of your life being angry at someone who repeatedly did something inconceivable to you? Perhaps you were abused as a child. Perhaps you were raped by a relative. Perhaps you witnessed a horrible occurrence that has stayed with you for far too long. What if, as a result, these events have held you back from emotional intimacy, vitality, or abundance? While no means an easy task, nor a quick fix, there is something you can do. You can do your life's work.

Choose what the meaning of life might be for you, and then take action. If you haven't figured out the meaning of life or your mission within it yet, you're not alone. Through repeated trial, error, and correction, let your mission come to you. The path to knowing can't be thought into existence. Let go of that through meditation and surrender, and all will become clear. What you'll likely hear is that by using your own special gifts, you were brought here to heal the hurt.

If you have been a victim too many times, you can remain feeling angry or hurt, or you can begin to heal. And one way to heal yourself is by preventing the same thing that hurt you from happening to someone else. If you have victimized others, you can remain feeling shamed or guilty or you can begin to heal. And one way to heal yourself is by preventing the same thing that you did to others from happening to someone else.

Burning karma, planting seeds—call it what you will—it is our job to learn from the past and do what helps others. But with all the conflicting ideas from various dogmas, traditions, and more, how do you know what is in the best interest of the people? This is determined by asking yourself: Does this help more than it hurts? Does it support my emotional and spiritual growth? Does this feel correct in my heart and soul, or is my Ego getting the best of me? What would happen if everybody did this?

✪ Reclaim your birthright of joy!

If you were raised in an environment of fear and conditional love that has made you feel small and unimportant, raise your own child's self-esteem at every chance. Teach your children that they are the love of Source made manifest, they make a difference, and that they can attain whatever they wish by being compassionate, loving, and giving more than taking. If you don't have children, raise awareness of what happened to or because of you, or offer a hand in an orphanage or a hospital for sick children. Join, fund, or start a foundation. Compassionate, selfless education and service can be a powerful step in healing your own deeper layers of pain and illness!

Without even realizing it (because giving feels so good), you are healing your own hurt by healing the hurt of others—we are all interconnected. When I had my awakening, I saw everyone and everything as jagged lines of color and energy against a black backdrop. Everyone was connected to everyone else and everything, directly or indirectly. Picture a spider's web where each of us is a small strand. Connected through time and space, if we open up to it, we can feel the joy of people thousands of miles away. We can also feel their pain. And often do, though subconsciously. Because of this connection, you can raise the vibration of yourself by raising it in others. How?

Always see them as not one step away from pain, but one step closer to health and their true magnificence. See them as not one step away from despair, but one step closer to joy. You can be the bridge to bring them there. With a smile, donation, hug, or by sharing where you've been and where you are heading, you will begin to heal the hurt, not only of yourself, but of all of those whose lives you touch, which, is of course, everyone.

CHAPTER 8

Are You Ready, Willing, and Able to Heal?

Are you ready, willing, and able to reclaim your health? Can you let go of those conditioned responses to get a glimpse of what's on the other side of pain or illness? What will you do without it? What would your life look like without the anger that's been holding you back?

Envision a perfect day. What would it consist of? Friends, work, play, challenges? Fine dining or a quick meal? What would waking up feel like? Would you embrace your lover before getting out of bed, or grumpily mope toward the bathroom while cursing the concept of mornings under your breath? Would you give gratitude to your higher power for the gift of life, make a gesture of love to it, and honor all that you see, feel, hear, smell, and taste? Can you let go of the to-do list long enough to feel the air go into and out of your body? Can you feel the arteries pumping fresh blood and nutrients to your cells before rushing off to work, or the post office, or whatever it is that you believe you have to rush toward?

Now, write out your perfect day below. Use some of those questions above as a guide if necessary. Go ahead; I'll wait. Stop reading, and do your assignment. Are you resisting? Are you sure you are ready, willing, and able to reclaim your health? Not enough room, you say? Then use the margins! Get creative. Come on now; get busy:

_____

_____

_____

_____

_____

_____

_____

Great job! How do you feel?

What? You didn't write anything?!?!?! Go back right now and write something. We'll wait. Okay, welcome back. Writing down your feelings, fears, and aspirations makes them more tangible; it's a checklist of what you want and no longer want, and perhaps a blueprint of what's to come. If you didn't know what to write, perhaps you're caught up in the mind that doesn't want you to get well. Your Ego would prefer you hang onto resentments. Is that what you really want? Many people are just unsure, even a bit scared, "What will my life be like without this anger?" Ask the Universe to show you the answers. You can't know what you haven't experienced. Be okay with that.

This may be difficult for some of you. Just remember that inherent in all of us is the capacity and desire to love everyone we see. For a gentle reminder: spend a few minutes with an infant. Remember that you were once that way, too. No matter what your school teacher, doctor, mother, religious instructor, or father said or did, ultimately, under all the layers of their own pain, in their hearts they have love for you. Only their hearts have been closed down due to their own pain in an effort, even if unconscious, to protect themselves. All too often, we close our hearts when in pain, but a better idea would be to ground ourselves and open up. Why? Because you're going to feel the pain eventually, so why not do so now. Purge the emotion before it causes physical problems.

Your ex-partners, even the ones who hate you or the ones that you hate, they too have love for you. If there is or was any passion at all, even if it is intense hatred, there must have been love at one time, but something made you or them close up. We are all love in motion. We only need to reclaim that innate state of being by going within our deepest selves and letting that energy burst right through our folded arms, shallow breath, closed chakras, and tightened muscles.

Once you are ready, or even as a method to become more open, try this exercise to purge yourself of both the frustrations of not being open and the stuck feelings that have led to ill health.

Begin by sitting quietly. Bring to your mind's eye the awareness that you discovered using The Five Steps to Health in Chapter 4. Recognize that you were taught, though indirectly, to hold back the ever-present love within you. Reclaim the love that is always around you by forgiving the mistakes of yourself and others. It is a cycle that will never end—until now—the moment of commitment.

Now, in this moment, begin to feel that the person who you feel anger toward is in pain themselves. Begin to feel the loss of someone you love who has left their body. Notice we are all on a path. Choose: Do you want to perpetuate this pain or begin the healing process?

Spread your arms wide and open up your chest to feel the heart open, too. Envision streams of anything that is not love leaving your heart, muscles, veins and organs. Give each painful feeling a color and a sound. Feel or scream these sounds out loud. Watch those colors go from a fiery red to a calming, soft blue, then to a warm summer green, on their way to a delicious white stream of love from your center. Then send that stream of love outward to everyone you used to think held you back, or who you used to believe disliked you, or who you used to think was evil. When you feel a tingle anywhere in your body, know that the Universe got the message, and so did you on a deep, profound level. Like a river before a man-made dam is installed, energy is healthiest when flowing freely. And so are we. When you feel heat where you used to feel cold, know that whoever you sent positive energy to has received it in whatever capacity they presently can.

✪ After about 15 minutes of doing that, **claim your birthright of joy**. Notice how your breath has changed and how relaxed you are. It's normal to cry or laugh, or emote whatever you've been holding back. Whatever happens, even if it's nothing at all, trust that at some level, something has shifted.

The next time you perform the exercise to become more open, add positive commitments: "I commit to becoming healthy," "I commit to expressing love," "I commit to showing forgiveness." With repetition, whatever you consciously say or think becomes rooted in your subconscious mind. Repeat these commitments with feeling, and not just casually saying them while, for example, watching *Wheel of Fortune*. Let them become a deeper part of who you are. Some people tap lightly along a particular meridian, or energy pathway, in their body to invoke the psychosomatic healing response while repeating these words. This further cements these healing mantras deep within. Even if you are unfamiliar with meridians, you can tap your sternum lightly and get the same effect.

In time, you will act and feel healthy, loving, and forgiving. Anything can become easy with practice, so why not practice something that will transform your health and life every day?

NOTE: *Not only does the body follow the mind, but the mind follows the body. If you assume a hugging position when mentally forgiving someone, it further amplifies the message. If you associate a yoga asana with a particular emotion or feeling, you can regain that feeling and reinforce healing just by assuming that asana! Notice what your body does in reaction to emotions. If you are feeling disconnected or sad, you may find yourself stooped over, looking downward, with arms internally rotated. If you stand tall, stay present, look people in the eyes and have your shoulders back (chest/heart energy open), your mind will recognize the change and alter your physical energy. Act as if, and the "if" will be!*

If you are having extreme difficulty, it may be that you aren't quite *ready, willing, and able* to heal. Perhaps you have repressed anger so deeply that you do not wish to forgive the other person. That's fine if that's how you are really feeling, but it is important to see that you are actually hurting yourself by doing this. By your being unable or unwilling to forgive and move on, you are keeping the resultant blockage (pain) in your body. Work with a trained, intuitive practitioner to push you because it's very difficult to do this on your own. This is no different from having a personal trainer or life coach help you overcome something you seem unable to do on your own.

Some of my clients think that without the challenge of their pain or illness, they won't feel inspired do the spiritual work to ascend to the next level. A logical thought but not a true one; that's the mind convincing you it's unsafe to get well. You can't know what it's like until you're there, and know that just by taking the journey others will be inspired by your messages of hope, Sharing your gift is the greatest gift you can give. If that doesn't get your heart pumping with excitement, close this book now!

It's time to look at your healthcare and see what has been working and what has not been working, given what it is you say you wish to achieve.

> *Holding on to anger is like grasping a hot coal*
> *with the intent of throwing it at someone else;*
> *you are the one getting burned.*
>
> —BUDDHA

CHAPTER 9

How to Release Regrets, Guilt, and Shame

How many of you have regrets about things you've done or said, or failed to do or say? How many of you have been taught to feel guilty for things you didn't even know weren't acceptable by someone else's standards? Most of us carry around the energies of regret and guilt, and they devour us. Rarely brought to light they stay in the dark, where they can only fester. What's brought into the light can heal. The most common physical manifestations of these disintegrative energies are a weakened immune system and when in the pelvis, sexual dysfunction. If you're always attacking yourself, and words have power, eventually you really will be attacking yourself way beyond what words are thought capable of producing.

People carry guilt and shame in their pelvis leading to painful childbirths.

"But wait a second, are you saying childbirth needn't be painful?"

Yes, I am. And not because I'm a male. I've given channeled, individualized visualizations and meditations to pregnant women. One said that by using the visualization, all it took was three painless pushes and she was done. In fact, a well-known medical doctor and women's health expert has said that the process can even be orgasmic.

"Now you've gone too far, Dave!"

We haven't even begun to touch the surface of what's possible. It's actually pretty normal if you step back for a second and think about it. On the physical level, a baby passing through the birth canal can stimulate the area known as the *Gräfenberg Spot*, or *G-Spot*—one of the most sensitive places that ignite sexual responses. Oxytocin helps with contractions and is released with nipple stimulation. And when a woman is relaxed and in pleasure, so is the baby. And the baby can exit in joy. What's more natural than that?

Guilt and shame stay in the pelvis and can lead to impotence, fears, infertility, lack of orgasms, and even sexually transmitted diseases (STDs). Were you taught that sex is dirty and that you should save it for someone you love? By believing it's dirty, what are you saying about life and relationships? There is nothing intrinsically wrong with sex, dirty sex, kinky sex, gay sex, or even sex with consciously applied pain. As long as two (or more) people are consenting to it, where's the harm? If you believe God will judge them, why would you waste any of your time or energy on what others are doing? He can take care of it if He feels a need to do so.

So who was it that taught you to feel guilty about the most natural acts in the Universe? People with little understanding of energy or what life can be about. Sex is the act responsible for each of our births. What could be more beautiful? Of course, if you believe that we're all born in sin, it may be hard to reconsider. As with all things, though, how something is used and the intention behind its use are what's needed to consider when debating if something works or doesn't work, as you decide what it is that you are trying to accomplish.

Recognize that it's only others' perceptions that you've decided to believe that can make you feel guilty. This isn't always easy to reverse, but it's true. We need to learn from the past so we don't repeat harmful behaviors. Guilt is a very powerful and destructive energy that is best released before major damage occurs. In fact, holding onto guilt and shame can lead you to repeating the actions you feel guilty and shameful about!

It's important to learn the lesson, then purge the energy, so it doesn't occur again. Beyond any lessons learned, the infinitesimal details of the past are best forgotten. Any regrets, *should haves* or *shouldn't haves*, guilt, and shame are a waste of energy and actually re-create experiences where we can once again be regretful, or filled with *should haves* and *shouldn't haves*, or shame ridden. If you are living in Regret Land, there are five powerful steps you can take:

1   **Recognize.** Recognize that you've been feeling separated from Source. If you were not feeling separate, you'd be seeing things from the larger perspective and would know fully that nothing happens by chance. All events, no matter how painful, are opportunities for growth. What you've done or failed to do are pieces of the perfect puzzle. Recognize your part. Take responsibility because no matter how painful, you called it forth.

2   **Expose.** Expose whatever behavior or situation that brought up regret, guilt, and shame to at least one person you feel safe with. What you conceal gains energy; what is brought out into the open is given room to be healed.

3   **Feel.** In a safe environment, fully feel both your regret and the pain you've caused another.

4   **Compassion.** Practice compassion toward yourself and the other person, no matter what. No one is perfect. We all make mistakes. But if we look at the mistakes and learn, they're not mistakes at all.

5   **Commitment.** Make a firm commitment to yourself, Source, the person you contacted in Step 2 above, and if possible, the person whom you offended. Apologize

from your heart for any discomfort your actions may have created in others. Tell them that you've learned what works and doesn't work and are committing to only doing what does work. If direct communication isn't possible with someone you offended, do it energetically. During a meditation, have this same conversation with their higher self. Visualize yourself speaking with them along with their understanding and appreciation. Trust they will get the message.

CHAPTER 10

Integrating Healing into
the Subconscious Mind

Healing with Source, Example No. 3

Mike was having difficulty raising his left arm over his head. Being a personal trainer, Mike had assumed the cause was a difficult shoulder press.

I said to him, "You're right *and* you're wrong. The shoulder press very likely aggravated the pain, but it was not the cause."

Mike became open to the possibility that there was an underlying weakness there to begin with. "People everywhere, including your clients of varied strength and size, are able to do this exercise and not experience pain. **What does this motion of raising your arm represent too you?"**

"Volunteering," he replied.

I asked him what he didn't like about volunteering.

He said that he wasn't feeling appreciated—that volunteering was not putting money in his wallet.

I asked him if he enjoyed doing the work he was doing for free.

He said yes.

"So, you're getting upset from not receiving payment for doing something you enjoy that you don't even expect to get paid for?"

I told him to think about this for a while. When I saw him a few days later, he was smiling widely. While swinging his arm freely, he excitedly told me: "I've been thinking about what you said, over and over, and by the second day I was pain free—so much so that I didn't even need to consciously think about my issues with volunteering. It became second nature to understand what I was doing to myself by having unrealistic expectations." Mike was able to do this because he was open to the possibility that thoughts are energy, and energy is creative. He accepted that he was the source of the pain and took responsibility to make a change. Mike utilized the most powerful healing that money can't buy; you can't buy what you already have!

Patience

When you teach a child how to walk, do you give up after a few tries? While watching them fall do you laugh out loud, saying, "Well, it looks like this one's not gonna get it—can you pass me the beer nuts?" More importantly, does the child give up? No way! How about learning to play an instrument? Did you quit if you couldn't reach your fingers wide enough to play a G chord? Within a few years, that child is running around you in circles and you're singing to her while playing a G chord with ease.

Do you remember the first few times you drove to your new job? You planned the route and on the way paid attention to certain landmarks. You made mental notes, "Oh, there's the health food store" or "Great, a branch of my bank is nearby." After a few trips, the journey there and back became deeply rooted into your subconscious—you barely had to think about it along the way. If you've ever driven somewhere and not remembered driving there, you know what we mean.

My brain? That's my second favorite organ.
—*WOODY ALLEN, COMEDIAN AND FILMMAKEr*

Integrating the concepts we've been talking about is no different: as each new concept is introduced, your brain creates pathways that remember this new information. It takes time to build the brain cells necessary to do just about anything consistently and without effort, especially if those things are replacing preexisting ways of being. By living the Five Steps to Health lifestyle, even a little bit each day, your energy levels will increase and you'll begin to feel better about yourself. You won't be in as much pain nor will you crave unhealthy foods. Your body will feel freer, your mind more open, and love will flow from you *toward* the people you used to expect it *from*.

> *But what about living free of pain and illness sooner? Is it possible? You say that energy moves at incredible speed, but what about for me? Can I alter my energy so that this neck pain will go away, or at least subside so I can do the work of awareness, acceptance, opportunity, gratitude and forgiveness without having my attention diverted to my neck pain? What about more serious conditions? Am I supposed to just meditate and be thankful because I'm not dead yet?*

Do what resonates with you in this book repeatedly until, during, and after you see results *along with* what your doctor recommends. If you've got a tumor, don't spend your entire life rereading this book and hoping the tumor will vanish in a few days because you've been forgiving people, repeating affirmations, or giving your money to charity to test the laws of karma. If you've separated your shoulder, don't spend your time raising awareness only. While centering your mind and breathing deeply can help reduce the amount of pain you are experiencing, have the doctor remove the tumor or set the shoulder—then reread this book and apply the principles. Your memories are stored deep within you, and it is often very difficult to release them on your own. Picture your life as a good book—each memory has its own page. Some pages barely contain scribbles. Others are overflowing into long, intertwining chapters. Each chapter builds upon previous portions. So it's okay if it takes a while to see results because it took a while to notice the problem that may have been developing over decades. It can take time and numerous visits to a practitioner for major shifts because some conditions are end results of several lifetimes. When you see this bigger picture, it's easier to accept the situation and have the patience to reverse it.

Self-Acceptance

But what if you've done all the steps described in this book but still have that neck pain? What if, after a few weeks you feel no different than you did before? It's real easy to give in to old habits and you may find yourself taking an aspirin or a painkiller and hoping that the pain will go away. Your doctor or even a friend may tell you that there is no mind-body connection, so you'll take mind-numbing prescription pills instead. Eventually you'll remember that you've been blocking the messages that your body is sending. There may still be a desire to go back to the pills because it is easier, but this book will still be in your home. Enjoy even this part of the process—*the process is how you learn*.

Whenever you learn a new language you translate those words into your current language to understand what it is you are studying. If you do that here you will never heal. This is about learning a new language that is not based on the old one, yet still evolved from it. It evolved out of necessity because the old methods are in need of updating—not because they don't work ("work" is subjective), but because there is another paradigm readily available.

Like a good yoga practice, you only need to go as far as you are ready to go. Each day you can attempt to go farther: the challenge lies with being okay with wherever you are. Criticizing yourself for not going farther, or telling yourself that you *shouldn't have to* do something or *should be able to* be something quicker, are keeping that negatively charged energy in place. Accepting where you are at in the moment is key to healing.

Life is a perpetual instruction in cause and effect.
—*RALPH WALDO EMERSON, PHILOSOPHER*

Do your best to monitor your thoughts. And if you don't, or feel you just can't do so regularly, try not to beat yourself up. Remember the baby learning to walk? This may seem paradoxical, and what if it is? Life as we are accustomed to perceiving it is linear, but in actuality it is cyclical. Life itself is a cycle of birth and death, rain and evaporation, and loving and having your heart broken. Even the earth and the stars are cyclical in their orbits and their very existence. Linear thinking is limited; cyclical thinking is multifaceted—the latter is where all the fun is!

Full self-acceptance of who you've been and who you are is often difficult to achieve. So, just how long have you been hard on yourself? A better question is "*Why* are you so hard on yourself?" It follows that you cannot begin to release self-criticism without an answer to the latter question. Do you think you were born self-critical? Did you get frustrated as an infant if you couldn't walk right away, or did you fall, laugh, or cry, and then try again?

Various authority figures make themselves known throughout your life. With humans being the way we are, what are the odds that you received the same information in the same way from numerous authority figures? You were very likely confused by all the conflicting messages, but they offered one common message: you were taught to feel wrong—or imperfect—in your mind and body.

If your teacher told you one thing and your priest told you something different, what is a child supposed to do? She will not know there can be more than one "right" because even at thirty—or eighty years old—few people recognize that possibility! It's a catch-22 where the student will be wrong no matter what. This is where you have created the energy of being wrong, and from those moments onward you have spent your entire life trying to prove everyone else wrong just to make yourself feel right! Two wrongs don't make a right, especially when the definitions of right and wrong are relative.

NOTE: *You will never be "right" because there is no "right."*

This is where defeatist perfectionism starts. You will always be wrong in your mind. That sets up energy patterns whereby you will not love yourself. You will then criticize yourself for being wrong, or for not attaining perfection. Even the definition of perfection itself is debatable! How can you ever achieve what you cannot even define!?

Recognize that perfectionism is self-defeating, and quite simply try again. Do this once a minute or once a day; it will not matter because all roads lead to the same place, anyway. The only difference is the speed at which you drive. Or walk. Or crawl. You only fell short and only did so *in that moment.* Invite yourself to re-create yourself anew in each creative moment called NOW.

CHAPTER 11

When Words Have
Too Much Power

We have not lost faith,
but we have transferred it from God
to the medical profession.
—*GEORGE BERNARD SHAW, AUTHOR AND PLAYWRIGHT*

It's common for us to give or receive tragic news poorly; we were never taught how to disseminate or receive it skillfully, and helpful tips on grieving usually aren't shared until after the loss is experienced—not the best time to learn something new. When doctors say, "I'm sorry, you only have six months to live," it's considered to be in the best interest of the patient and the immediate family, but knowing the power of words, how many times has someone's life been shortened—or lengthened—by what might be called an externally placed prophecy?

Someone may be too ill to hope to recover, and as sad as that can be, who gave anyone the right to say something that definitive about an unknown future? When a psychic predicts the length of time you have to live he or she is considered a lunatic, but a doctor is rarely questioned. This is not to put down medical doctors; it's just a reminder that the power of words can have a deadly effect. People's beliefs often create their reality, and words from an authority figure are often taken as gospel truth.

Perhaps a more loving and honest way to convey information about a terminal illness would be, "I'm sorry, you have advanced X. I've seen persons with similar symptoms live for a few months, and I've also seen some live much longer." If it really seems like death is imminent, they could even add, "In the meantime (I hate that word; time is not mean!), why not live at the highest level you can, taking each day as a gift? Take each moment to clean up all your unfinished business and share your knowledge and experience with those who will listen."

Patients may be able to inspire others with the same symptoms, and because of the intrinsic and therapeutic nature of sharing and compassion, patients might actually prolong their own life, or at least improve its quality while still here. It may or may not aid in long-term recovery (there are too many factors to take account of to know for sure, and certainly too many to list here), but without trying, you'll never know.

Your doctor groups together your symptoms and categorizes them within a known informational field. She classifies you according to your symptoms based on those of other persons, and labels you with "X" or "Y" "syndrome" or "disease." While this may be effective at times, it reduces overall efficiency because there are too many factors un-accounted for. For example, if there is a study done in rural Italy on stress, how does that have anything to do with persons who are stressed in New York City? Likewise, a nu-tritional study done in Kenya will yield different results than one done in Canada. You may not really have "X" or "Y" "syndrome" or "disease" — merely similar symptoms.

Once you are told you have a specific disease, you are subject to its preexisting treat-ment and cure rate—which may or may not be conducive to healing. There is more to health than a diagnosis and a medication! Once you are given a specific diagnosis, you become part of collective unconsciousness and its understandings of a particular disease. Kierkegaard said, "If you label me, you negate me," meaning that once someone or something has been named, it, he, or she cannot be anything else. If I address this symptom of pain as something completely different than your medical diagnosis, for example, "a misalignment in the quantum field of pure potentiality," I am no longer subject to the laws of collective unconsciousness. This frees you to experience a reduc-tion or elimination of the symptoms in a dramatically lesser period of time. Given the right circumstances, along with a leap of faith, thoughts— therefore energy, therefore matter—can be transformed. We can realign the quantum field of pure potentiality!

Other practitioners can implement this theory should they choose to. It is my belief that many practitioners could assist the body in curing itself relatively quickly if both she and the patient agree it is possible, regardless of the actual treatment given. If you are dubious about a quicker mode of healing, you may experience a longer recovery time. If I tell you exactly why you have this pain, and you do not believe me, it is prob-ably only because your Ego has convinced you that you need to be right. Being right might make you feel good about yourself, but you will still have the pain. Because each person is unique, I may be able to help Felix and not Oscar, even though they may have what appears to be the same condition. There are too many variables to put a one-size-fits all technique out there and expect it to be helpful for everyone. The cookbook technique, which is what we've already been doing, has limits; therefore, it has only moderate success.

Oy Vey! I've Got a Bad Back . . .

So, you've got a BAD back, a BAD shoulder, or a BAD knee. Now ask yourself, *What did this back, shoulder or knee do to warrant such a negative label?* Knowing what we now know about the mind-body connection, what are you telling yourself about these lovely parts of your body that have been so good to you until one or more of your thought processes changed all that? I invite you to call each area of pain or discomfort you are experiencing *healing*, not *bad*. At a lecture, an attendee said she reduced her pain in just a few minutes by changing her vocabulary! You can do it, too!

Focus on a positive vocabulary. Words have vibrational power, and as they are used, the energy associated with them affects you. Catch yourself when complaining, blaming, or feeling like a victim. You may need to do this every minute or once a week. Consciously choose to accept responsibility, then create the circumstances necessary to heal and enjoy your life. This book is filled with many ways of doing so, but in the end it's only words. You have to make these words come to life. You have to live these messages of better thinking, positive vocabulary, awareness, and forgiveness until it becomes a natural state of being. It may take time, but it works. And there are no side effects or a lifetime of office visits. It doesn't cost a lot to be real in your thoughts, word and deed. But it costs you a whole lot not to.

CHAPTER 12

Let Go of My Ego

We will now go back to the beginning of time, which, by the way, never occurred. Time is a creation of the human mind—time is cyclical and vertical, not linear and horizontal. There is only one moment, and it is called now. Time could never truly begin, because to say that also implies that it will end. But for the purposes of informing rather than confusing with metaphysical psychobabble, Earth and its inhabitants are in a never-beginning and never-ending cycle. Because we are made of energy, all of us were never created or destroyed; we've merely gone through many transformations!

THIS particular incarnation of Earth (did you think that only people can reincarnate?) has certainly seen its ups and downs. The story of Noah and the Ark was a parable for a time, much like our own, when technology outgrew its inhabitants. People didn't have the spiritual awareness or level of consciousness necessary to contain and effectively use the technology being created. Indeed, a global warming did occur that wiped out much of the planet.

While the continent of Atlantis was buried under water, some of the people of that time escaped because they understood how things truly work. Their wisdom was passed on; it's held within what Jung calls the "collective unconscious" and can be accessed by sixth-sense capabilities, which all of us possess. You have to choose to develop that skill, just as you would with anything else you wish to learn. It can take time, but what a fantastic use of time, don't you think?

Ocean water, some eight millennia prior to the aforementioned time, was drinkable. Water seeks its own level, both physically and energetically. My own intuitive work with Source has taught me that the high quantity of salt in ocean water today is an end result of the collective tears both physical and energetic from uncountable numbers of people throughout all ages. Grief has become ingrained in our lives. The healing of our own grief and that of the collective needs to become a primary goal for all of us.

As we begin the healing process, something else makes itself known that must be understood in order to move forward on our path. Metaphorically, it is a doorway that we need to walk through in order to consciously reach the state of bliss that is our birthright. The door that separates our conscious reality from this bliss can be understood as a metaphor for our Ego. It cannot be seen, but we have all felt its effects. While it has been written about over the ages, the door separating us from the Creator is most readily understood through metaphor and parable. The best known and perhaps the most accessible of such writings can be found in the Christian Bible, but there are many spiritual books that seek to explain this esoteric concept. In Aramaic, an original language that was spoken some 6,000 years ago, the name for Ego was pronounced *Sah-táhn*, or Satan. Satan, or Ego, is the *internal*, intangible force responsible for keeping us in check. Its job is to make sure we do not get too cocky. And with good reason.

The Creator knew that we could manifest anything we desire—including health—once we knew we could, so She gave us what any good creator of any great game would—an opponent! Why? Because if we could win every game and manifest anything at will without an opponent, there would be no challenge and no sense of accomplishment. Boredom would settle in very quickly. Life would have no sense of purpose or direction.

We think that being the winner is the ultimate goal but that's a fallacy. If at the beginning of the basketball season someone were to hand Michael Jordan the championship trophy and the Most Valuable Player (MVP) award, saying, "Here, you're only going to win it all anyway," do you think he'd accept? Would he just want to be handed the championship, or would he want to enjoy the challenge of attaining it through his own hard work and skill? Indeed some of the reasons Michael Jordan won the championship so often were his passion for the game and enjoyment of the challenge. He wanted to guard the other team's best player, and he also wanted the ball at crunch time!

> *You may find, that after a time, having is not such a pleasing*
> *thing after all, as wanting. It is not logical, but it is often true.*
> —SPOCK, FIRST OFFICER, USS ENTERPRISE, STAR TREK

I've seen similar behavior in the animal kingdom. A dog will drop a tennis ball from his mouth to chase another one thrown just a few feet away. Joy does not reside in the having; it's in the quest! If this quest in getting what you think you want is a chore, how much do you think you'll enjoy the fruits of your labor? Is it worth many years or even decades of torment just to make your first million dollars? Unless the process is fun or at least a challenge, it will be emotionally empty, and you will be driven to make your second million dollars, thinking that a second million will make you happy. But it won't. It's a vicious cycle when not seen for what it really is. If you view the journey as an opportunity for growth rather than a burden, not only will you attain your goals quicker but the fruits of victory will taste sweetest.

The thrill of victory can only be properly felt if there is a worthy opponent. Most of us will not have the opportunity to test ourselves in a high-level sporting competition, like Michael Jordan in the NBA championship, so for the rest of us, the Creator arranged our very own internal opponent: the Ego. Many people seem to want to declare war on the Ego, declaring that its dominance is the reason our lives are such a mess. This, of course, is exactly what any intelligent opponent wants—he or she knows that the more energy you give to it, the stronger it gets. The only way to defeat the Ego is by loving it into submission! Picture it like a small child trying to get their way. You wouldn't declare war on a child with whom you had a disagreement, would you? If that child were upset and began to cry, you wouldn't hit them, would you? Okay, some troubled and misinformed parental figures might do that, but their actions are precisely those that what will lead to that child then becoming "a troubled child." Ideally, if a child is sad, you'd hold her and let her know she's safe, letting her know that she's free to be herself. Think, then, of the Ego, as a small child of sorts. It believes it is you, and it wants its way at all costs. And it will do anything to get it.

> *Pay attention to what you're thinking—and you are not your thoughts.*
> *Your thoughts are created by a tiny, tiny little group of cells about the size of*
> *a peanut sitting in your left hemisphere, and many of us let that little peanut*
> *rule our lives. And you have to recognize that it's just a group of cells that*
> *is designed to tell stories so that we feel safe in the external world… So pay*
> *attention to what you're thinking and then decide if those are thoughts are*
> *creating the kind of life you want to create, and if it's not, then change your*
> *thoughts. It's really that easy.*
>
> —*DR. JILL BOLTE TAYLOR, NEUROSCIENTIST,*
> *ON OPRAH'S SOUL SERIES*

When we realize the Ego is responsible for certain actions and behaviors, it is both easier and more effective to coax it into submission with love than to deny its power. This takes a lot of time and discipline, but the benefits of doing so are life-altering. With a reduced Ego, we can better communicate with truth. We can align ourselves to the flow of life and totally accept its many directions and forms. Peace of mind leads to peace of body, which leads to a feeling of connection to others and to the spirit world, which leads to vitality, freedom, and joy. If you didn't just yell out loud, "Sign me up!" then put this book down and go channel surf.

There are several ways to reduce the Ego's power. One is awareness and appreciation that this is the way things are—that the Ego is not you, nor are you solely the Ego. Understanding this, with practice, you can start to become proactive rather than reactive.

Proactive behavior recognizes truths and takes a moment before reacting. It means using the soul to make informed decisions rather than the Ego, which makes automatic, reactive ones.

A typical example of reactive behavior is experienced when another car cuts you off. The reactive mind gets angry and takes the event personally. It may even desire revenge. But this is what feeds more of the same: you cannot fight fire with fire and expect not to get burned. A proactive mind takes a moment to think and maybe even ponder the possibility that in the back seat of that car is a pregnant woman who needs to get to the hospital as soon as possible. But our Ego takes things personally because that's its job! We have two choices: we can gently ask it to step aside, using our love and attention, or we can give it energy by seeking revenge on a driver you don't even know! The choice, as always, is yours to make.

One of the best tools for training the mind to be proactive is meditation, which naturally reduces the Ego's grip on your thoughts and actions. It makes you aware of the moment and, after a time, trains you to respond from that place of compassion and understanding as opposed to vengeance.

Your Ego will sense that you desire its demise, so it will come up with any excuse for you not to better your life. From "Oh, I don't feel like going to yoga class; it's too cold out" to "I can't meditate correctly. My mind is too active to sit still. I'm not a yogi living on a hill in Tibet who's unconcerned with paying bills, romantic relationships, and traffic." Guess what part of you is speaking then!

By the way, because I am an "expert" and you're not, I am naturally so much better at getting rid of my Ego than any of you are!

Ha! I love that joke!

Ahem.

But seriously, folks…

Appreciate the Ego for what it is and know that you don't have to hate it to win the game. Picture you and I playing a game of chess against each other. You don't have to hate me to defeat me. In fact, by creating that kind of negative energy, you're only affecting your own health as well as affecting everyone around you in a negative way. It's a downward spiral. Even in a sport like boxing, fighters who perhaps are brutally beating their opponent know that their opponent is not their true enemy, just a temporary adversary. Nothing can ever truly be won with hatred.

Oftentimes, because the Ego is so good at providing distraction, you need a support group or friend with whom to practice new concepts. I recall crossing a street and spotting a brand new Corvette passing in front of me. My desire-ometer went up to a 12 on a scale of 1 to 10! My girlfriend at the time, who was deep into meditation from a Buddhist perspective, asked me, "What part of you wants that car?" I immediately knew what she meant—that it was my Ego speaking—and my desire for the Corvette was gone instantly! To this day, I can admire a Corvette from afar, yet have no desire to own one. It's a lot more sensible to drive something that doesn't insatiably drink gasoline while screaming, "Hey look at me!" The latter is the mantra of the Ego.

How many of us have believed for a time that we could lose those extra 40 pounds, make more money, and find the perfect partner just by following the steps so cleverly outlined in a book or workshop? You truly believed that this was the time for your ascension to the next level of your life, and after the workshop you were so excited that everyone around you wanted a piece of what you appeared to have. Some of them inquired and followed through, but most went back to their daily routine, and after a time, so did you. Ever wonder why?

The answer, as you may have already guessed, is within you. It's your own built-in opponent, the Ego that feels its potential reduction or even demise, and like any entity instinctually would, imminently cranks itself up another notch toward self-survival. It will present to you the most compelling reason that will most effectively sabotage your newest endeavor. But instead of recognizing what's truly occurring, we have too often given in and taken time to verbally beat ourselves up. We're our own worst bully.

But when you recognize which part of you is the bully and which part is the truth, you can more effectively monitor your thoughts, words, and actions and know what's truly best for you. You can actually step back with the conscious mind and be proactive. Once you recognize it is the Ego at play, you can take steps to reduce its grip on you! Even better, take those steps ahead of time so the task won't be so difficult when it arrives. Prevention is truly the best medicine! Clearing the mind in advance gives better access to truth as opposed to our own internal and mostly fictitious mind ramblings.

Imagine you're in sixth grade and the school bully is kicking you from behind when seated in the classroom. You react and he sees he's getting the better of you. He's bigger and meaner, so you don't dare fight back, but you do live in torment each day and he knows it. His Ego is getting more energy from your misery. At one point, if you truly surrender to the situation and really see that he's in a lot of pain, your natural tendency to cower will be reduced. He'll stop bullying you because his Ego isn't getting what it needs any longer from you. This is what is meant by *turning the other cheek*. You can consciously choose to understand that it's his Ego and not the true person that is doing this. It's time to see the bigger picture and exercise compassion. If someone is looking to antagonize you, make a conscious, loving choice not to play that game.

Perhaps you have a family member or colleague that seems to thrive on controversy. I call him, Anti-Man. Whatever you say, he has to disagree. I once heard a conversation that went like this: "It's cold out." And Anti-Man replied, "No it's not." Temperature is subjective, and this was a 70-degree day. For one who was used to warmer temperatures, it seemed cold. But Anti-Man had to say it wasn't. Imagine if the conversation began, "I feel cold." Think about the difference energetically when someone just states how they feel. It's tough to argue with that approach, so when dealing with your own Anti-Man, try to focus on "I feel . . ." statements and watch what happens.

While Anti-Man may not necessarily be mean, his Ego is in charge and gets a kick out of proving itself right. And your Ego is likely to respond with a similar energy. But if you can truly see what's going on, you needn't play that game anymore. By being proactive, you can easily say, "You're right, thank you," even if you don't really mean it! Watch what happens when you can do that! He's likely be too confused to continue.

Once while I was working in retail, a customer was yelling at my boss. My boss ran around the counter and imitated the customer, yelling toward where he himself had been standing behind the counter a moment prior. The customer was so surprised by this tactic, and perhaps saw what he looked like, that he stopped yelling. When you do something out of the ordinary, the other person's Ego does not know what to do. Egos can freeze, and hearts can thaw. Any relationships can mend as long as we don't let them go down a negatively charged spiral of Egos fighting other Egos.

> NOTE: *There is no such thing as a mean person—only people who do not know how to handle their own pain.*

To overcome the negative effects of the Ego, you need to decide that you're not going to entertain its messages any longer. So, how do you know it's his voice and not yours? How do you distinguish the messages of the Ego and those from your heart?

If doing something only serves the self, the message is from Ego. If doing what you think you hear seems to hold you back from challenges or increases separation from others, it's the Ego. If on the other hand, it feels right in your heart, and the message is about awareness, connection, unconditional love, or being of service for others, then you know it is the true you.

> *Whether it is right or wrong, thinking makes it so.*
> —*WILLIAM SHAKESPEARE, HAMLET*

Of course if you have no belief in such a system, all of this will be irrelevant to you. I hope, though, that by book's end, you will know why both opinions are right and will have no desire to put down what you don't agree with. Because that's what we tend to do: if we disagree with something, we are quick to judge and label it wrong. This keeps us safe and our paradigm unchallenged. However, "wrong" is merely an arbitrary term for *something you do not agree with.*

88

Ultimately, none of this means anything, unless you want it to. Nothing is right or wrong intrinsically; that is, in and of itself, nothing means anything. Even "nothing" when broken down reads, "no thing!"

When the Ego notices you are better able to ascertain the difference between the his words and those of sprit/soul/Source, he'll get angry with you and try to trick you into getting his way. He'll pick on you and call you names like unlovable, unattractive, or unworthy of success. And because he knows your weaknesses better than anyone, his advice will seem logical! So you'll veer from your chosen path. You may even go on a downward spiral of negative feelings and emotions for days or weeks or more. But if you're attentive, at some point you'll be reminded that you can win this game. Pat yourself *on* the back as opposed to stabbing yourself *in* the back. Step away from reactive behavior and begin living proactively. Until you know it's a game, and until you know the rules, you cannot possibly win.

A few of my clients had been diagnosed with bipolar disorder. While I do not address that *per se*, I can address the symptoms and help provide clarity through intuitive, verbal consultation. They possessed a similar characteristic. They were extreme people pleasers. Their Egos had convinced them that to be liked they had to always do for others at the expense of the self. They were not accepting of themselves as fully human—did not allow themselves to have feelings of anger or even dislike toward other people or themselves. What you resist persists, and the so-called negative aspects, or our shadow selves, were bottled up so tightly that eventually they had to burst! This caused extreme fluctuations in mood and even lack of discernment as to who was talking, the Ego or the true self, thus the unflattering label.

It is totally normal to dislike something. It is unhealthy to pretend to like everyone and everything. Not only does it lack integrity, it will only make others dislike you; moreover, it takes too much energy to live that way. Author Debbie Ford says that it's okay for some people not to like you; some already don't, and you're just fine!

I can dislike you and still love you, meaning I accept that we disagree on say, politics, or even what to put on our pizza. But I support your choices and your desire to be you. To practice the highest vibrational energy, that of unconditional love, means to accept others and yourself as they and you already are.

We all have these Ego-driven lower self-vibrations. Given a certain set of symptoms, many of us are capable of doing what we'd never think possible. Look up the Stanford Prison Experiment, for example, where peaceful college students were abusive to other peaceful students within two days of being given absolute power in a mock prison. This is one of the reasons we should never judge anyone. We can never know what's possible until we're in a given situation. Until we walk a mile in another's shoes we can never truly know what it's like. After the experiment ended, one of the "prisoners" was asked what he would have done with that power. Seeing how other equally peace-loving students could become so vile so quickly, he hesitated and said, "I don't know."

Most of us like to believe we're incapable of harming another, but if someone were attacking your loved ones and you had the means, you would most likely do whatever is necessary to protect them. The human psyche is vast and complex; to only accept the parts you label as positive is draining at best. One can never find and develop the true self without embracing the entire self, including egoistic thinking and all. It may not be pretty, but it's human. The alternative is living like a Vulcan—and even though they are so stoic and logical, Vulcans go crazy every seven years. (I know many of you think that *Star Trek* was only a television show. My Ego has informed me that if you think that way, you're just living in denial!)

When your Ego makes its presence known, give it a tangible existence. Maybe even name it. I named mine Hugo (as in "you-go" here, "you-go" there).

Raise your hand next to your head as if you're wearing a hand puppet. Invite him to ramble about your inadequacies and fears. Then, place your other hand on your heart, warmly look at Hugo, and invite him to gently go away. Say to him, "Thanks for your suggestion, Hugo; however, I am going to listen to my heart now." Then place your Hugo in your pocket to symbolize what it is you are intending to happen. If you need to do this every minute, hour, or afternoon, so what. You've nothing to lose. And it can be done anywhere. If someone asks what you're doing, just tell them "Hugo has a big mouth, and I needed to calm him down." And then they will either ask for more information or think you're nuts. If the former, you may have made their day. I guess that could be true in the case of the latter as well. After doing the puppet exercise for a while, you'll find you won't even need to actually act it out as the clear intention takes over. With practice, anything can become an automatic way of being.

Our Ego has convinced us that we cannot win and that we are all separate from each other—and none of it is true. For many, the Ego has worked magnificently well—so well, in fact, that we identify with it so totally, we don't even believe it has a separate existence inside our heads. When we realize, accept, and then work through this challenge, we can then see our true selves emerge. You experience yourself at a whole new level. Others react to you differently. As your mere presence begins healing others, they want to be around you more. Those people who used to bother and drain you no longer do. You feel lighter and have more energy! That is the true self reemerging!

The true you is unconditional love. Know this, and everything will change.

If Wanting To Be Right is Wrong, I Don't Wanna Be Right!

If you believe or if you don't believe, you're right!
—ANTHONY ROBBINS, MOTIVATIONAL SPEAKER

Proving ourselves right is a national pastime. How many know-it-alls have you met? They are everywhere. Heavens, some Smart Alecs even write books to demonstrate how knowledgeable they are. (But not this author, of course!) Seriously, though, how many people can really be an expert on everything? Why do some of us need to show mental prowess whenever possible? Perhaps this stems from getting positive feedback for being what your teachers labeled "smart."

> NOTE: *Intelligence is often confused with the ability to memorize, agree with, and regurgitate what you are told.*

Traditional schooling teaches us that "smart" is good (A's and B's on our report card gets us presents and love), but not knowing something is bad (C's and D's might get "What's wrong with you?" energy). A good education teaches us how to think. Much of our current system might get us on a trivia-based game show or fit into the status quo, but it more than likely won't directly help us invent anything new.

The desire to be right (or the fear of being wrong) is so prevalent that many of us meet new concepts with intense resistance. This is why we consistently maintain behavior that leads to disagreements, poor relationships, even wars, and never seem to learn from our mistakes. It is only when we step outside ourselves that we understand what is really happening. Although this is simple, it's not easy.

The kind of intelligence that is transformative begins in *daring to ask why we need to know* that "the sin of 30 is one half" in trigonometry class. Transformative intelligence lies in *daring to ask why* history books rarely if ever describe the opposing point of view when teaching about war. Or *asking why*, as read in the Bible, God chose to help only one side and smite the first born male child of the other. Weren't they just innocent children?

By taking an honest look within and around you, you will soon see that the old habits of living no longer serve you, and you will eventually aspire to newer habits. Once you get over your fear of change, things will flow effortlessly. Change is the essential process of all existence. The quicker you embrace this concept and reduce your fear of the unknown, the quicker you will manifest your dreams.

Even if you're on the right track,
you'll get run over if you just sit there.
—*WILL ROGERS, HUMORIST*

You can follow esoteric practices and think that everything will come to you if you are coming from the right space—that of love. Indeed, many of the Eastern teachings can be interpreted as meaning just that. That's great if you can live without any money, or are willing to renounce all those things you are accustomed to having in your life. In the United States, if you have only the right mental attitude but don't do anything to support that belief, you'll find yourself homeless pretty fast. So why is it that we hesitate to make changes or do anything new, when it is obvious that our old ways are not getting us what we want? Sometimes, it's in our perception of learning.

Everything you've learned in school as "obvious" becomes less and less
obvious as you begin to study the universe. For example, there are no
solids in the universe. There's not even a suggestion of a solid. There are
no absolute continuums. There are no surfaces. There are no straight lines.
—*R. BUCKMINSTER FULLER, ENGINEER, DESIGNER, AND ARCHITECT*

If someone said to you, "Hey, come with me to a great self-help program," what would be your typical reaction? Even if your friend has the best intentions in mind, you may take the invitation personally, thinking, "What's so wrong with me that they feel I need to do that?" What if they asked you to join their multilevel marketing company before you asked about it? Or even told you not to mix fruits and proteins because that would weaken your body's ability to digest well? If you are like most people, you will initially shun anything new because it doesn't fit your belief system.

The main dangers in this life are the people
who want to change everything or nothing.
—*NANCY ASTOR, FIRST FEMALE MEMBER OF PARLIAMENT*

It is rare for children to have positive memories of learning because they are continually told what to do, what not to do, how to behave, how not to behave, and *what* to think instead of *how* to think. When you are scolded for not learning fast enough or given grades of C's and D's in school, the Ego convinces you that you must be "less than" other people: "I am less than she is because she got an A," or "I am less than they are because I cannot pronounce the *th* sound well," and so on. If you believe any of these long enough, it becomes real to you. You really start believing you have less capability than another person and, therefore, may adapt a "Why bother?" mindset. "Why bother if I can't do it well?" "Why bother if I'm going to fail anyway?"

The fear of not getting it right, where *right* can be merely an opinion of a given authority figure, will hold you down and prevent you from taking any chances, yet risks are where all the fun is! You can pursue certainty all you like; it's comforting to know that when you step on the gas, the car will go forward. It's great to know the quickest way to travel between points A and C. But too much certainty in your life will become tiresome or even boring. There is always a need for variety in anything we do. Maybe you can drive down a different road, or get from A to C while stopping at B just to notice the difference. But most of us don't. Why not?

We need to look at our perception of learning. Become aware that a particular action or way of being you've associated with learning is no longer serving you, and then take steps to rectify it. This is done by recognizing that your perception of learning, like everything else, was something you were taught or even made up years and years ago. Likewise it can be changed by choosing to see the joy in the challenge. You will feel better when you do.

NOTE: *A way to get over your conditioning is to understand what it really is. It is merely the continuation of a thought pattern that has yet to be questioned: "Is this working?"*

If we want to create anything new, we'll need to admit and even welcome the possibility that there is something we don't know. Without this honest look at the self, we are solely behaving and relying on our Egos. If we do this, our lives will stay the same as they are now. Take a course, read a book, have a conversation with an expert in a particular field. Do anything to keep your mind growing.

Denial is Not Just a River in Egypt...

This above all, to thine own self be true.
—*WILLIAM SHAKESPEARE, POET AND PLAYWRIGHT*

Many people deny that a change is needed, or doubt that it can be accomplished. They hold onto tradition from long ago and never look to see if what they're doing is working in the long term. Even Pope John Paul II kept up with the times by changing some traditions that may have been more than a thousand years old!

What are we in denial about? Go into the dating scene for just a moment. Denial is everywhere. People deny they are still in love with their former partner. Some deny their age or real occupation. And with online dating, there's no way to know that "Candy, the 21-year-old Hooters waitress" is really Herbert Finkelshwartz, the aging accountant!

I'd rather be hated for who I am,
than loved for who I am not.
—UNKNOWN AUTHOR

Say what you mean and mean what you say. Just don't be mean. Telling untruths will catch up with you. Many of us don't even realize how often we adopt an attitude of pretense. Spend one day telling only the truth, if you want to test this for yourself. If someone asks how you are doing, tell them how you really are feeling instead of nonchalantly saying, "fine," and see what happens. They did ask, didn't they?

Why are we in denial? Because we can't stand to think about the truth. Denial is a protective mechanism designed to hide us from our feelings. We live lives of pretense to avoid anything that might be unpleasant.

Most things we choose bring us closer or farther from one of the two extremes of pleasure or pain. Millions smoke, drink, or do drugs to deaden the perception of things that are too painful to deal with, and some just engulf themselves in activities that temporarily put the mind on hold, such as watching television, overeating, and playing in cyberspace. If that's what it takes to get someone through the day, then so be it; for everything there is a purpose. Yet your body already knows how much to eat and what—and it will let you know, too—if you are more mindful of what and how you are eating. Doing so will better allow you to listen to its innate wisdom.

Problems begin, however, when the need for instant gratification outweighs all else. This is a sign that Ego is winning the game. Getting through the day becomes trudging through the week, and that turns into dreading the upcoming month or even year. Imbalance occurs, serving as a catalyst for a long downward spiral in your health. While Western medicine may call this an addiction, I am choosing not to use that word. The power of words is such that if you believe you are addicted, you also believe there is little way out and allow yourself to become a victim, a convenient way not to address the problem. Try calling it, instead, *an unhealthy, learned behavior that can, in time and with patience and love, be unlearned.*

NOTE: *To reduce the craving for external gratification, it is best to see a qualified professional who understands the mind-body connection and can help guide you through a process of becoming more complete with yourself from the inside-out.*

When we notice that all of these blockages to happiness occur because of a rampaging Ego, we can take steps to calm it. We can see burdens as opportunities and seek higher-vibration persons with whom to associate. We can challenge our own minds to learn and grow into the next greatest vision you could possibly have of yourself.

The effects of not using our bodies for a while are very visible: obesity and muscle atrophy. The impacts of not using our mind in a healthy way are less visible but are detrimental—we just don't see them until it is too late. When you learn something new, your brain creates cells and pathways that remember what you are learning, and when cells and pathways are not used, they deteriorate. Stagnation equals death of the mind, death of fun, and the death of life. A possible end result of not utilizing the wonderful gift of learning enough—not stimulating the mind—is the disease known as Alzheimer's. If you've always wanted to speak Spanish, or learn how to cook Spanish foods, *¡ahora está la época de tomar una clase!*

CHAPTER 13

The "True" Self

The Ego is not the "true" self. The true you is a sparkling diamond deep within. It's like a highly polished brass urn—a sparkling vessel holding unconditional love deep inside. Similar to the genie in the bottle, once you rub the outside and open the top, out pops the magic. The urn's shiny surface is practically blinding, but it begins tarnishing the moment we are convinced we are no longer connected to the Source.

Our spirit comes from a vast realm and chooses to inhabit a baby's body upon conception (I've worked with many women who've had an abortion and was able to channel that the spirit of the baby was either already happily reincarnated or a spirit guide for that woman—none were sad and none were angry at their mothers). The spirit inside the fetus is nurtured for nine months. At birth it is often greeted with a spanking, then separated from the only human it's ever known—sometimes immediately—for hours or more at a time. The umbilical cord is just long enough to allow breastfeeding for a reason. Separation anxiety begins when the cord is cut. The urn begins tarnishing in that moment. And grief is born.

Behavior Modification Gone Awry

Q: Have you ever wondered why so many people have issues expressing love as adults?
A: Because children are taught to repress their feelings from early on!

From Day One, we respond to our children's actions with reward or punishment based on our own judgments of what we believe is acceptable. Babies learn that crying gets them a bottle, whining gets them a toy, and yawning gets them rocked to sleep. Crying doesn't *always* mean that Baby is hungry or that something is wrong, but we get nervous when a baby cries and project upon them our reality. We mistakenly think they must be sad and believe they need to be rescued from feeling bad.

Everybody was a baby once. Oh, sure, maybe not today, or even yesterday.
But once. Babies—tiny, dimpled, fleshy mirrors of our us-ness that we parents
hurl into the future like leathery footballs of hope. And you've got to get a good
spiral on that baby, or evil will make an interception.
—*THE TICK, SUPERHERO*

Some children learn that acting out gets them a whack on the bottom. If they cry too much, touch things they don't understand they should not, or even walk too far away from their caretaker, some children are spanked. Like preaching abstinence to those with natural, developing hormones, this is behavior modification theory gone wildly astray. We're actually creating the exact opposite of what we are hoping to create. By stuffing their mouths with a pacifier when they cry, we teach them oral satisfaction as a deterrent to communication. This could lead to hand-to-mouth addictions, for example, overeating, smoking, and alcoholism later in life. By slapping them on the bottom when they are merely expressing curiosity, we teach our children to repress their desires and emotions, and they learn that violence is a proper way of dealing with what is really a misunderstanding.

Caretakers, relatives, and even strangers respond to children's initial vocalizations and laughter with more vocalizations and laughter—all positive reinforcement. Yet a few years later, a child often sees that all those sounds they made as an infant that got them all those laughs, hugs, and kisses are now perceived as annoying! Children then are either told directly or just assume on their own they are to be seen and not heard. Sometimes that warning is given in the seemingly harmless expressions, "bite your tongue" or "bite your lip" coming from a well-meaning schoolteacher or babysitter.

While I do not specifically recall those being said to me, I did develop symptoms later in life as a result of that mindset. At 28 years young I developed painful sores in the mouth, which were diagnosed as apthous ulcers. Almost a dozen well-meaning medical doctors and practitioners of holistic chiropractic, acupuncture, and spiritual healing didn't help. Years later, I realized the ulcers developed when I wasn't speaking my truth! I also had to forgive those practitioners toward whom I felt anger and frustration. What a wonderful if not painful message that was only made much more painful by my ignorance of what was really happening— all the more incentive to write this book.

So, what's a child to do after receiving all these conflicting messages? Sometimes they become shy. They feel judged by others and rather than go through the humiliation of having their words ridiculed, judged, or just not understood, they quite naturally minimize talking. And this makes sense, for if you're living as if you're walking on eggshells, then why would you want to take another step? Sometimes this manifests as a low speaking voice, a closed-down posture, or mumbling. The way to overcome the barrier of shyness in your children is the same as prevention: love them unconditionally for who they are, as they are, when they are. And always listen more than speak.

Think about your own childhood. All you ever really wanted was the approval of your parents. You wanted to be told and shown that you are loved—faults and all. Right? Do you think your children are any different? Or your parents, for that matter? I assure you they're not, so give them what you yourself wanted, and you will receive what you so fervently desired. It is an unbreakable karmic and energetic law!

> *Wise men (persons) talk because they have something to say;*
> *fools, because they have to say something.*
> —*PLATO, PHILOSOPHER*

Alternatively, the child may become an attention seeker. Oh, you know the type. If this need is not dealt with early on, years later he will seek the attention of anyone in earshot at every opportunity. He will be "in your face" about everything, constantly looking for that positive or even negative reinforcement—merely wanting acknowledgment. This individual must make sure you hear him and if you do not recognize him quickly enough, the attention-seeking activities will increase. He'll continue until you recognize him, even if your form of recognition is saying, "Shut up already!" Adults who never questioned this methodology often grow up believing that acting out for attention is a normal thing. Ultimately, all people want is to be recognized. Is there any reason for someone to stop this behavior if it's subconsciously validating their existence? So, what to do?

- Babies who lack the cognitive ability to speak can learn sign language. In fact, my friend's kids could sign before they could speak. I sat in amazement watching them sign to indicate they were hungry, wanted more of anything or that they'd had enough!
- Let your baby cry. They'll let you know if it's something serious or if they are just getting more air into their bodies. You'll be able to feel the difference, too, by quieting your own mind and just being open and present. Often, they'll stop within a few moments and will be fine.

Some time after birth, the infant begins to sense that something else has changed. As the baby grows older and others call her by her name, she starts to experience life as her own person. "Oh, I am Wilma, and she is Mama!" and "That is Dada, and I am still Wilma."

Wilma seeks that oneness again but finds herself limited in movement. And all of these thoughts help form and solidify the Ego to protect us from the pain of separation. Additional forms of loss continue—a lost toy, friends who switch schools, parents divorce, and so on. Either way, Wilma's body knows what's best and most natural to heal the grief—Wilma begins to cry. A beautiful thing.

Some infants cry for another reason altogether. They don't know that they and you are separate. If they feel that you are upset, in pain, or ill, they can actually take on some of the burden for you. This is why babies, who lack the ability to create pain or illness with their own thoughts, worries, or fears, can develop symptoms of pain or illness—indirectly and, of course, subconsciously. Many do not realize this empathetic response even later in their lives and continue to have an unhealthy connection to their others. They're called too caring, or develop what is known as sinusitis or asthma. Some become lost in a path of endless therapies looking to heal old wounds that aren't even theirs, wondering why they're not feeling better each week.

As an adult we can give back those pains, and as brutal as that sounds, we are actually helping the other person to complete that individual's mission! It is better for all involved in every way, but it is often a difficult cord to cut because you have been bound by it for a long time and are now wondering what will become of Mom or Dad if they are given back their grief. They will be fine; odds are pretty high they won't even notice any difference. What are a few raindrops in an ocean of plenty? If you feel more comfortable, surrender and ask spirit to take on their burden for you. Either way, it is imperative for your own growth to realize that *metaphysically, no one is responsible for the soul of another person.*

Do not—ever—tell your child, "Be a good boy and keep Momma happy" You are imprinting way too much responsibility on their young lives. And, in most cases, children will believe their perceived sense of responsibility because parents and other adults often let their moods be swayed by the actions or inactions of an infant. Babies see the connections: "If I'm funny and cute, they all laugh, and when they laugh they seem happier" or even worse, "If I cry they get upset. Sometimes they hit me. They can't see that I'm just purging grief. I just want to be loved."

> NOTE: *This crucial time is often the target of my sessions, which involves going through and releasing grief. We go back in time and tell that baby that he or she is loved. This changes the neurochemistry of the individual and assists in healing grief-related physical and emotional ailments.*

Prior to fetal life, each soul is one with everyone and everything. Just a thought can bring the soul to any time and place. In fact, time and space do not exist as we currently understand them. Think of the soul in this timeless realm as the Queen on a chess board in a world of only chess boards—no limits! When the soul chooses to join a fetus, the soul still feels at one with *all that is*, only *all that is* has now changed. All that is, now, is its mother. This is when the fetus can actually pick up on and be affected by the physical states of its mother. We know that if you smoke, it's as if your baby is smoking as well, but what most people do not think about is how anger, fear, and grief of the mother affect the fetus, too.

All emotions either produce or alter chemicals in your brain. And these "emotion chemicals" quite obviously can affect the fetus as well. When pregnant, more than ever, think good thoughts and trust you will do the best you can. With tools like this book, advice of experts, and an openness to what truly is, you can have happy, healthy babies. You can also learn from other cultures that know about and recognize the physical, energetic, spiritual and emotional aspects of premature separation, and, therefore, do not distance their young so quickly from their mother. They also feed the child *before* he or she gets too hungry.

Energetically, the fetus not only picks up on the thoughts of its mother but of everyone around her. So it might be time to add energy work or spiritual counseling for the family to your Lamaze or underwater birthing classes!

Nothing that grieves us can be called little:
by the eternal laws of proportion, a child's
loss of a doll and a king's loss of a crown
are events of the same size.
—*MARK TWAIN, AUTHOR*

Having once tasted it, we crave the state of wholeness—the connection with Source that we had prior to birth. We mistakenly believe that other people and things are there to bring us back to a state of wholeness—our true self—but that's not possible. Other people and things are our guides and teachers of this painful lesson: you are never alone unless you think—or are taught—that you are!

As years go by, everything you and others do confirms the perceived separateness. In most people, the Ego is insatiable in its role of protecting us and helping us fulfill our desires. So, we begin to seek that wholeness in every possible way. Some get glimpses of oneness in a relationship and attempt to use that vehicle to complete themselves, but it never works. There is always something perceived to be missing, and that something is the awareness of the true self and the true connection with Source. As we reconnect with Source, we'll attract better situations and people, and have more energy to unconditionally give to all our relationships!

As we go through life, we experience other people—seemingly separate entities—leaving us. They'll move away, break up with you, and some spend too much time without you—for example, at work or with friends. All of these separations are departures that can produce feelings of loss and subsequent opportunities to grieve. Of course, at some time, you will experience the loss of someone as they leave their body. And, because you were taught that death is the end of everything—an afterlife of eternal condemnation—you once again grieve. We even grieve when we believe our loved one is nestled on big, puffy clouds where everyone wears white and plays the harp (I'd grieve even more if that were true—that sounds like hell to me!).

Do you recall hearing, "Big boys don't cry!" or "There, there, little girl, everything is okay. No need to shed tears."

WELL, IT IS NOT OKAY TO HEAR THAT!!

We are often told "don't cry" when grieving. Others say this because they don't want to see us, their friends, sad. Sadness is normal! The release of emotion needs to be supported not stifled. Often, just having someone being there for you is more important than anything they can say. And it's okay to let them know this: "You don't have to say anything. Just remain present with me in this time of need, that's all." Who would say no to that?

We must teach our young and show by example that it's okay to cry. Grieving is a powerful, healing energy, but when it is repressed, problems develop in our health. Be it allergies; lung conditions; difficulties with our body, hair, and nails; or even dry skin, releasing grief will prevent all of these and many more. Grief affects the pancreas' chemical production, leading to a propensity toward obesity. If you're not eliminating well (large intestine/colon issues), have ear problems, or even get diagnosed with depression, it is the repression of grief energy that is very likely the cause. One must learn as soon as possible that grief is a friend, not a sign of weakness, and we should let our friend be seen. And heard.

It is time to foster a child's sadness, not repress it. If they learn to repress it, they will also repress other emotions. Not only will they be afraid to express grief, anger, or fear, but they learn to repress their humor, joy, and love as well! I find it ironic that I used to feel it was horrible to make another person cry; now people pay me for it!

Between the expressions of laughter and weeping
there is no difference in the motion of the features
either in the eyes, mouth or cheeks.
—LEONARDO DA VINCI, ARTIST

All negative memories and repressed emotions form scar tissue on the aforementioned brass urn that holds our true selves. The healing process sometimes involves gently scraping the tarnish from the urn like a lead pencil that's gone outside the coloring lines, and other times we need to painstakingly scrape it off, layer by layer, inch by inch, or mile by mile, to once again see and feel our purest light. Spiritual growth is the process of removing the scars to let the true self shine! The process isn't always pretty. It will be very different for everyone. But this process is quite beautiful, and so are you. This inner beauty becomes more obvious as your true self is awakened. You live in integrity and authenticity and do so with ease. You are shedding layers of emotional garbage to let the true self be seen and heard.

The mind commands the body and the body obeys.
The mind commands itself and finds resistance.
—ST. AUGUSTINE, PHILOSOPHER, THEOLOGIAN

Because emotions are repressed from Day One, expressing and releasing them is sometimes uncomfortable, even painful. But only because we have resistance to feeling them. If you were totally open, there would be no pain in the release, and everything would be purged easily, but few people are that open. Think about and allow yourself to feel the grief that's been lodged in your body for so long. Sometimes, movement is required, other times breathwork, sometimes both. Layer by layer you can shed the grief, even if it hurts. That's why emotional healing is tough to do on your own. At the first or even second sign of discomfort, many people distract themselves from going deeper. It's best to work with a practitioner who understands this process and can push you through the emotional wall.

Why would you want to do this?

Because it's the ticket to freedom.

I've worked with people who have lost weight, cleared allergies, reduced symptoms of what are referred to as colon issues, and regained energy and enthusiasm just by holding space and allowing them to feel what's been locked up for so long. It's tiring holding all that emotion in, even unconsciously. Once it's released, there is healing and a new zest for life!

The process of healing old emotional wounds won't always be painful. I've done many sessions where Source comes in and releases it for you. I tell everyone to be open to whatever happens. It's all effective, but we have to release our expectations and attachments. We need to trust that what happens occurs for our best interest, and that it's what we are capable of handling in that moment.

On rare occasions, laughter commences. At one workshop, I was laughing to the point of gasping for air while a good friend was crying her eyes out in intense pain as she recalled old painful memories. The dichotomy was odd as my inner healer wanted to reach out and share my joy with her, but the practitioner leading the event said to stay within the self. Fits of laughter that lead to tears are as healing as a good cry. The destination is the same; the difference is only in the process. There are even laughter yoga practitioners who would concur! Dr. Bernie Siegel, author of *Love, Medicine, and Miracles*, says, "the more the humor, the less the tumor!" Real or faked, laughter can release enough endorphins that make morphine seem like bubble gum.

CHAPTER 14

How to Get What You Really Want (Aruna's Chapter)

To give pleasure to a single heart by a single act
is better than a thousand heads bowing in prayer.
—MAHATMA GANDHI

One look and I knew she was special. I introduced myself. She said she was from India and in New York City for just three days. Her name was Aruna.

"Three days? Is that enough to get to know someone and get married?" I joked.

Aruna laughed, "There are plenty of available women in this country for you."

We conversed some more. It was obvious I was talking to an enlightened woman. She was an ear surgeon, here to attend the funeral of a family member. I commented on how respectfully she treated everyone, her warm demeanor and accepting, almost "knowing" glances.

"That's because everyone is beautiful." Aruna said.

She added that because she saw everyone as already perfect, whole, and complete, the reverse occurs. Others saw her that way, as well. This, of course, made sense; yet, who does that consistently? We all slip back into judgments now and again, but it didn't seem like she ever would. Wondering how she learned to live this way, I asked if it was cultural, economic, national, or religious, and she simply replied that it was who she was. Later, when Aruna said she's gotten everything she's ever wanted, I asked for the secret . . .

"I never have asked for anything for myself."

"Huh?" I replied.

She repeated her statement: "I never have asked for anything for myself."

Growing more inquisitive, I asked: "Is prayer a part of your daily routine?"

"Yes, very much so!"

"Then you do pray for things for yourself! You must be praying for abundance, happiness, peace of mind, clarity."

"No, never, not once," she replied.

"But you seem abundant and happy." I said.

"I am" Aruna replied.

"Hmmm... Do you pray for your patients?"

"Yes, always. I ask God to take me before taking any of them. It has never failed. Everyone I've ever operated on has fully recovered."

Aruna had mastered the law of getting what she really wants. How is this possible? She knows that we are all one, that we are all a part of the same energy system called the human race. She knew experientially what many of us have only read: that when you do something for someone else you are doing it for yourself as well.

However, there are times when we must take care of our own needs first. You can't take care of others at your own expense. Giving is not always better than receiving. In fact, that's an old myth created by those who only wanted to receive! So, like all things, balance must be attained. If Aruna hadn't gotten proper sleep the night before her surgeries or kept up with the latest medical information, her patients may not have been so fortunate. Knowing this, she takes care of herself well, too.

Take care of yourself first, and know that giving begets more giving. If you pay for your friend's movie ticket with no thoughts of why or what you might get back, the next time you're out your friend will probably buy you something. Maybe they'll splurge for the $12 size popcorn. If either of you spends a little more, it is irrelevant. It's the fact that you are giving that is important.

> NOTE: *To give in this way is unconditional, like love when practiced at its highest vibration. Unconditional expressions of giving and loving release attachments and give life to that which was once dead.*

Give, but don't seek your own self-worth through helping others. Give because you want to. Because it feels good. And never give out of pity. For example, it is better to offer someone a job than to give him money. The latter will create dependency on you and others. You are very likely power-tripping on feeling noble or pious. At the same time, this will never allow the other person to grow emotionally or spiritually. It is always better to teach self-empowerment. People who are dependent on you will never learn responsibility. Some will continue to ask you for favors of time, companionship, or money. Eventually you will resent these requests, even though you might not know *why* you're feeling resentful at that time. What a waste of energy! To be of service in general is wonderful and can warm the heart, but to overdo it and create dependency damages everyone involved.

Flatter me, and I may not believe you.
Criticize me, and I may not like you.
Ignore me, and I may not forgive you.
Encourage me, and I will not forget you.
—*WILLIAM ARTHUR WARD, NEWSPAPER EDITOR, AUTHOR*

Walt "Clyde" Frazier, the Basketball Hall of Fame guard of the New York Knicks, said that when people on the street ask him for money, he instead hands them his business card and instructs them to call his office for assistance in getting a job. Clyde then added that none of them ever do. By doing the enlightened thing, he is offering the best kind of service one can give—an opportunity for them to become self-sufficient. But the beggar likely sees himself in the role of a victim. Stuck in old patterns, he finds it difficult to do something to improve his life.

…you give a beggar 50 cents for free,
And the beggar says,
"Hey, if that's all you can spare,
You need it more than me!"
—*SAM CAMUS, SINGER/SONGWRITER*

We can survive without taking from others. We can give and empower others. We can be open to receiving what the Universe wants to give us. When we only want to help and advance ourselves, as survival of the fittest mandates, it is greed at its worst. It is greed that leads to: haves and have-nots, economic crises, starvation of entire groups of people, ethnic cleansing, territorial disputes, wars, and large businesses making millions of dollars by polluting Mother Earth. Survival of the fittest is short-term survival. Nothing more. Because it may have been apropos in the past (or useful in the animal kingdom) does not mean it must be apropos for humans today. In the long run, greed is self-defeating. It destroys us and our planet.

Bobby Benson: [*indicating grave marker during a visit to Arlington*] That's my father. He was killed at Anzio.
Klaatu: Did all those people die in wars?
Bobby Benson: Most of 'em. Didn't you ever hear of the Arlington Cemetery?
Klaatu: No… I've been away a long time. Very far away.
Bobby Benson: Is it different where you've been? Don't they have places like this?
Klaatu: Well, they have cemeteries, but not like this one. You see, they don't have any wars.

Bobby Benson: Gee, that's a good idea.

—FROM "THE DAY THE EARTH STOOD STILL", GOLDEN GLOBE AWARD WINNER
FOR BEST FILM PROMOTING INTERNATIONAL UNDERSTANDING, 1952

When the long-term ramifications of any actions are not taken into account, it is the very definition of the lowest vibration of human selfishness. An obvious example would be drilling for more oil at the expense of the environment, whereas funding and finding alternative sources of energy would be better in the long term. Aruna exemplified this concept beautifully. She has the insight to see beyond the basic survival of herself. She is led by the concept of *survival of the most cooperative*. By taking care of others, her wants and more come to her through divine intervention, or Grace.

Beyond The Law of Attraction

Why do some people get all the things they desire? Are they smarter, wealthier, or happier than you or I? Maybe yes, maybe no. What they know is that through intention and the Law of Attraction, they can more easily sample life's delicacies. By focusing on what they do want as opposed to what they do not want, they can manifest just about anything! Makes sense, right?

But there is another secret that can speed up the process of manifesting what you desire—something only true masters regularly do. It is a proven technique for closing the window of time in relation to wanting and having.

Right now, on a separate sheet of paper or on your computer screen, make three columns. At the head of the first column write, "What I want" and list all the things you want.

Then, at the head of the second column write, "Why do I want this?" Then answer that question for each thing in the first column.

Now, at the top of the third column write, "How will I feel when I have it?"

Look at what you've written. How long have you been wanting those things in the first column without much success of achieving and getting them? Or if you had success, it was only temporary, right? Now look at the second column. How many of you have personal reasons for wanting things, as opposed to wanting things for the good of those around you? Would Aruna ever do that? Ask and answer once again, "How long have I been wanting these things without success?"

Now look at the third column. This column holds the secret of the masters. Masters know that feelings vibrate on a much higher level of energy than thoughts and even words. And the vibrations of feelings create reality much faster than words.

Imagine what it feels like to be able to over-tip with no financial fear. You are now sending out vibrations of wealth! Think about and feel what it would be like to hold in your arms your soulmate. You are now sending out feelings of unconditional love! Likewise, if you can feel what it would be like to be respected, understood, heard, and accepted, what do you think that vibration would send out? What you send out is what is returned!!

When doing the work in this book, intersperse the purging of negative energies with the thoughts and vibrations of what you really do want! Pull out the weeds AND plant new seeds. Do the former about an hour a week with a practitioner and the latter whenever possible. Do you want unlimited energy, more flexibility, or even extreme health? Imagine and then truly feel within you what it would feel like to be vibrant with complete range of motion! Then watch what happens!

The semi-physical analogy is that everything we want is in an emotional and energetic waiting room, or escrow. Let me explain:

Place your hand out in front of you, arm fully extended. Imagine this hand as a representation of everything you've ever wanted, the perfect job, vibrant health, whatever. Now see the area between your head and that hand as the opponent (remember that's the Ego). As we do our spiritual work, the opponent loses energy. And because nature abhors a vacuum, once the opponent is weakened, everything you've always wanted is not only clearly visible, it comes to you almost effortlessly. Manifest in this way, and you're bound to be happy. Do it the old way and no matter what you wanted and even attained, you'd likely be miserable, still wanting more and more. You have to know what it is that you truly want and why. When you know the *what* and *why*, then the *how* makes itself clear to you. The above exercise probably showed you that you want to be happy more than wealthy—and now remember that *happiness is a choice*.

> *Happiness is when what you think, what you say,*
> *and what you do are in harmony.*
> —*MOHANDAS K. GANDHI*

Happiness is not something that is attained from another person, place, or possession. If we look outside ourselves for happiness, we are bound to be unhappy. We have to *choose to experience happiness* in each moment, the Now, no matter what is happening externally to us.

> *The happiness of life is made up of minute fractions—*
> *the little, soon-forgotten charities of a kiss or smile,*
> *a kind look or heartfelt compliment.*
> —*SAMUEL TAYLOR COLERIDGE, POET, PHILOSOPHER*

Happiness is attained by releasing control of the future. The future is merely an idea and cannot be controlled. Therefore any thoughts of doing so are a waste of energy that is usually manifested in the forms of worry and anxiety. How to rid the self of anxiety? Change your perspective of time. When we've released the regrets of the past and the attempts at controlling the future, we have surrendered to the present. And if you look around your present, personal space, the Now isn't too bad, is it? It could always be worse. Of course, we can plan for the future, but it is important to release the attachments associated with our plans.

Great spirits have always encountered violent
opposition from mediocre minds.
—*ALBERT EINSTEIN, PHYSICIST*

Others will listen to you speak about your newfound happiness or your process of raising awareness, and some won't get it. They may seem angry with you. This is *their* fear of change; don't take it personally. People have always put down what they do not relate to. Use this as an opportunity to love unconditionally! We spend so much energy worrying about what others think of us, it's amazing we have any left to use for other things. Don't let their stuff get in your way. Of all the quotes I've shared in my practice, psychologist Abraham Maslow's "Learn to be free of the good opinion of others" is the most powerful when it comes to this concept. Notice he says *the good opinion*, not *any opinion*. Just imagine how freeing it would be to live this way. Now stop imagining and live it. It's my belief that if you're in touch with your intention, and you know it is a benevolent intention for yourself and others, what others think is irrelevant.

✪ Reclaim your birthright of joy!

I don't care what you think of me. You have no power over what I think of me.
I know I'm as big as the universe—because I've been there and done that.
—*DR. JILL BOLTE TAYLOR, AUTHOR, ON OPRAH'S SOUL SERIES*

When attempting to create this new you, manifest a new job, or anything that other people see as living outside the norm, try to confine yourself to talking about your passion only with those people who will support you. Surround yourself with people who love you unconditionally. If you do not know too many people who fit this description, it is time to stop requiring from another person what they cannot give, do, or understand, and for you to learn what unconditional love means. It means, very simply, to let others be whoever they wish to be without judgment from you.

Those who say they love you but do so conditionally are actually judging themselves *through* you. There will always be someone putting their "two cents" into your life, and often with the most positive intentions, but those who understand unconditional love will discuss things openly and guide you to see your own truth. They will guide you to your own highest state of love based on what you say you wish to accomplish. When you can love unconditionally, others will feel this new you and return these feelings back to you. As you live this way, other unconditionally loving souls will make themselves known. It is a law.

NOTE: *If you judge everything people say to you, they will stop saying anything to you at all.*

Be Careful What You Ask For . . .

You train others how to treat you by how well you treat yourself
—*MARTIN RUTTE, CONSULTANT*

Our thoughts go out into the Universe and affect everyone and everything. And approximately 80 percent of the roughly 60,000 thoughts you'll have today are the same ones you've had for days, weeks, or even years. Thoughts are creative and our cells are mental warehouses, so what would happen if you thought "I am unworthy of love" even 20 percent of the time? You will be unworthy of love, even though no one really is. You will have thought yourself into believing it. Others will pick up on these thoughts and will actually treat you as being unworthy of love.

Have you had several short-term romantic relationships, constantly searching for the *right one*? Well, the right one is exactly who you drew to you! You may even draw abusers to you to fulfill the victim mindset you've created. That may seem frightening at the moment, but bear with me. Remember, you are learning a new language.

At some point in your upbringing, someone said something and you took it personally. Your father said he was tired after a long day at work and that he didn't want to play, and you thought, "I am unloved by my father," and it stuck with you. Your friends didn't want you on their basketball team in elementary school and you took that to mean you were unworthy of their friendship. Your mom was busy at her job and you took that to mean she didn't love you. Odds are against any one of these people taking the time to explain what is really happening because in their minds everything is already clear. Your dad really was just tired. Your friends really just didn't think you were that good at that particular sport, even if you were great at everything else. Your mother really was working because she needed to or because she wanted to, not because she did not want to be with you.

These types of occurrences set up patterns that we use to run the rest of our lives. Feelings of resentment or abandonment occur and reduce our ability to trust another person. We keep others at arms' length and never get close to them or let them get close to us. We may fear others doing something to bring up anger in us or even just get up and leave with no reason as to why. The beliefs we have now are thoughts about ourselves that we decided were true when we were barely old enough to understand what truth is. This is how the mind plays games, only up until now you didn't know it was a game. And if you did know that, you may still be searching for ways to win.

> NOTE: *In your mind is where all the insecurities lie. And that is the truth: insecurities LIE!*

Insecurities are not the truth. They are random interpretations of what you once randomly decided upon! YOU made it all up! It is time to take back what was once rightfully yours. You were born out of love as love, but your conditioning made you forget that. Not that you actually became what is not love; you only thought that you did.

Your boyfriend broke up with you in junior high school because he liked another girl. You took his decision personally and made it mean you are ugly and that you are unlovable. This stayed with you and now you're in your thirties wondering what went "wrong" because you are "still single." This might lead you to "settle" for someone who is "good enough" while you continue feeding the pattern of unworthiness. Even while in a relationship, you may feel unhappy but will have no idea why.

At that point it is common to look outside the self for answers. "If he can't love me, then maybe someone else will." After a time with a new partner, you will begin to again feel unworthy because you were looking to him or her to fill that void in you, and that is impossible.

> NOTE: *Unworthiness expands its grip on our freedom every day we do not see it as a prison from which we must break free.*

Process this new awareness and realize it no longer serves you. Release the feelings of unworthiness by recognizing that everyone is worthy of love, simply because it is our birthright; it is what we are made of. Your deserve-ability rating is always a 10!

✪ Reclaim your birthright of joy!

When I think with my mind, I seek answers to my questions.
When I feel from my heart, the questions dissolve into answers.
—BETH JOHNSON

Know the following: When in a bind, if we can quiet the mind, the best answer is always given to us. We can reclaim our worthiness by connecting to Spirit, for it is always there to guide us.

When we connect to Source, eventually we see the perceived unworthiness as false and will no longer take the abuse of others but forgive them, because we can. We do so because we know that forgiveness does not mean letting someone off the hook; we forgive them because we know that by harboring all that disintegrative energy, it will eventually harm us. We forgive because we understand that individuals do what fits their reality at that time, and you now realize it doesn't have to be your reality. You forgive by *canceling* the effects this person or situation has had on you because you know better. You forgive because you love yourself too much not to do so.

NOTE: *The shaman's technique: while waving both your hands across your heart chakra in alternate directions, say out loud, "Cancel; cancel."*

The Law of Infinite Possibilities

There is no better (teacher) than adversity.
Every defeat, every heartbreak, every loss
contains its own seed—its own lesson on how
to improve your performance the next time.
—OG MANDINO, AUTHOR

The Law of Infinite Possibilities dictates that if you're a musician pursuing a recording contract, be open to playing in a house band, on a movie soundtrack, or even in the subways. By being open to all of the infinite possibilities, you will be playing music for a living, but just not exactly how you planned it. Who's to say that one of these alternatives won't lead you to a recording contract? By having no attachments to the *how* in getting to a desired end result, you will also avoid disappointments. And disappointment can only occur when you have an attachment to someone or something being a certain way.

NOTE: *Everyone is a gift for you and you are for them as well. Feel-imagine living this way. Those who were once annoying become angels. Those who we used to find rude merely remind us what we do not wish to be.*

The Emotional Rollercoaster

How do you know you are evolving? When you spend less time thinking about, and therefore giving energy to, time spent that you are down. If you tried something and it didn't work out—if you fell short at a certain task—remember that life is an emotional roller coaster. We wouldn't understand the highs without experiencing the lows.

Picture your life as an on-screen heart rate monitor such as those you see in hospitals. When we're alive, it's beeping and moving up and down. And when we're dead, it flat-lines. This is true with life, as well. We too often get annoyed with the intermittent ups and down, but remember the alternative. Flatlining is death.

> *After all these years, I am still involved in the process of self-discovery.*
> *It's better to explore life and make mistakes than to play it safe.*
> *Mistakes are part of the dues one pays for a full life.*
> —SOPHIA LOREN, FILM ACTRESS

Many people try to live an even-keeled life to avoid any chances of being hurt, but re-moving the parameters where fear exists also removes any chance of experiencing bliss. The amount of time spent "down" on yourself will decrease as your soul evolves. If, for example, you had plans that fell through at the last minute, didn't make *People* Maga-zine's "50 Most Beautiful Faces" list, or just missed the train, you are only temporarily experiencing downs. Actually, the exact detail of what brought you down is irrelevant; when living in AWARENESS, this downtime is decreased exponentially. Staying in the down state is merely the conditioning kicking into effect—which you can choose to alter.

What about Failure?

> *It must be born in mind… that the tragedy of life does not lie*
> *in not reaching your goal. The tragedy lies in having no goal to reach.*
> *It isn't a calamity to die with dreams unfulfilled, but it is a calamity*
> *not to dream… it is not a disgrace not to reach the stars, but it is a*
> *disgrace to have no stars to reach for. Not failure, but low aim is the sin.*
> —DR. BENJAMIN E. MAYS, MOREHOUSE COLLEGE

What does *failure* mean, anyway? A more empowering way of looking at it—one that is more conducive to your emotional and spiritual growth—is to replace the word "failure" with the idea of "falling short." Words have power and calling yourself a failure under the old definition is damaging to you and your health. Don't believe me? Say, "I am a failure" several times in a row. Okay, now say, "I fell short" several times in a row. Which feels better? Examine why you fell short, make an adjustment, and try again.

> *I have missed more than 9,000 shots in my career. I have lost almost 300 games.*
> *On 26 occasions I have been entrusted to take the game winning shot. and missed.*
> *And I have failed over and over and over again in my life.*
> *And that is why I succeed.*
> —*MICHAEL JORDAN, FORMER NBA BASKETBALL PLAYER*

CHAPTER 15

Relationships and Soulmates

If our emotional lives could be represented by a letter, for most of us it would look like the letter C. The goal of the soul is to be whole, though, and filling in that open area of the C metaphorically results in the letter O. So we might think of the open area of the C as the missing piece from the puzzle of life. We'll do just about anything to fill in that space; yet, most of what we do fails to complete the circle. In fact, more often, we tend to soften the solidarity of the existing parts of the C, sometimes so much, to the point of becoming an… I

You'll C what I mean shortly.

Most people look outside themselves for answers. They'll take every workshop available, read every book in sight, and spend their lives in search of a destination; financial, physical, a great relationship, and so on, when the missing piece is actually spiritual in nature. The soul enters the body as an individuation of the greater whole. To attain the unity once again requires work in the spiritual realm, not just the mind and body. Ultimately, all we really want is the sense of reconnection—the feeling of safety and joy we had before we were born. As impossible as it may seem, there ARE ways to know that feeling again, here in our earthly incarnation. Purging what no longer is true for you and embodying compassion and unconditional love for others increases our spiritual awareness and the feeling of wholeness. When we see others with *Grandma eyes*—the look that shows she loves each grandchild equally—we give them the gift of our presence. Both you and they are better for your actions and the C begins to fill in and become a complete circle, an O.

Constant kindness can accomplish much. As the sun makes ice melt,
kindness causes misunderstanding, mistrust, and hostility to evaporate.
—*ALBERT SCHWEITZER, PHILOSOPHER, PHYSICIAN, AND MUSICIAN*

It took a number of years, but I learned that physical soreness and exhaustion after a full day of giving massage therapy was a choice—albeit an unconscious one on my part. Eventually I saw that by taking the self out of the equation, I needn't experience pain or even exhaustion at the end of the day. When I dropped my concerns about how well I was doing, or worrying if the client was enjoying the experience, or how much I was getting paid (or IF I was going to get paid when billing insurance companies!), I no longer felt sore or exhausted at day's end, but invigorated!

"O" people rarely get sick. Why? Because they are balanced in the mind, body, and spirit triune, and that is a precursor to optimum health. They understand that pain can be a friend, an opportunity, or a reminder; therefore, they do not fear it, knowing that fear will create it. They know that having pain does not mean they have to suffer. They understand that their immune system is capable of handling most pathogens and do not let angry thoughts get in the way and weaken it. They don't project, prejudge, or hope to change people, but love themselves and others as they are.

"O" people's concept of love is different. For "O" people, love is unconditional. They will never tell someone that they are good or bad based on their grades at school. They will never stifle the exploration of a child or tell them they are smart only if they do a certain thing a certain way. They will never tell their significant other they cannot do something. They will support any decision made by another; realizing it is just their part of a much bigger path. They will wear their learning like a pocket watch and only speak when asked. They will never force their will upon another person.

O Say, Can You C?

Communication is different for "O" people: they know it is how we listen, not what we say, that is most important. We often listen intermittently, interjecting our own opinions and judgments (to the self or even out loud) before the other person is even finished speaking. Notice your typical listening patterns—they are intermittent at best. Then for a comparison, watch another's reaction when listening attentively and without judgment—as if they were giving you the secret to life—even if they're talking about the most mundane subject you've ever heard. They will feel this openness you've created and feel more comfortable sharing their deeper selves. Spiritual wholeness requires improved mutual understanding. Among the ways you attain this is to improve your listening skills.

Silently keep in mind the following as you listen to others:

Your wisdom is great, and I wish to hear every word before it should strike the ground. Speak softly and slowly that I may breathe your words as your thoughts become my own.

As you listen to another person, try saying to them: "I want to make sure I understand you, so I'm going to repeat what you said in my own words, and you can tell me if I've understood what you're trying to communicate."

Breakdowns in communication are the primary reason that many relationships between lovers, friends, families, and business associates fall apart. How can any relationship be successful if you do not openly communicate with that other person or group? It will be like any episode of just about any sitcom, but it won't be cleaned up by the half-hour's end. Energetically and ethically, it is better to talk *with* someone than to gossip *about* them.

If Anyone O-bjects, Speak Now…

Unconditionally loving relationships are without needs. Needing something or someone is the surest way to push them away. It puts tremendous pressure on the other person to tell them they are the glue that holds you together. What would happen if they left? Would you really fall apart? Who could live up to that kind of pressure of completing someone? It is better to be a *counterpart* to someone; where they are an adjunct that elicits joy in you.

No one can complete another person or life, but that expectation is embedded in our current definition of a relationship, and it is sorely in need of an update. Perceived needs appear to go unmet, and resentment builds because eventually we realize that the perfect partner to complete us is a myth.

Two out of three marriages end up in divorce, and three out of four of divorced spouses remarry, only to divorce again. The problem lies in continuing with the same behaviors and expecting a different result. As with many traditions that are handed down blindly by older generations, we have to draw the line here and now. We marry for all the wrong reasons, considering what it is we are trying to accomplish, and we still expect things to work out. According to the statistics, they don't. Marriage "worked" when the human lifespan was around 25–30 years and a partnership was necessary to survive. Each partner had their respective jobs to do, and survival was a team effort. But today and in many countries, your basic survival—relative to caveman days, at least—is practically guaranteed.

The idea of marriage is a beautiful one when it is not encumbered with all the leftover rules from centuries ago. The joining of two persons can be a joyous adventure, but as it's currently defined there are too many expectations and attachments to the results. These attachments take away from the beauty of the journey. The many stipulations based on outdated ideas are best viewed as conditional loving. Any love that is conditional will be resented because it is the nature of the soul to be unlimited.

Successful marriages do, of course, exist, but they are predicated on your personal definition of a successful relationship! In the metaphysical view—or that of unconditional love—a successful relationship is defined by the purposes of mutual support, mutual spiritual growth, and mutual emotional growth, more than its length. Even a two-year marriage can be successful if it has been mutually supportive. At the end of the two-year period, if one partner has outgrown the other—and it is recognized by both parties—where is the harm? If a partner wishes to grow elsewhere or with another, it is not always an insult; however, we've been conditioned to believe it is, and we all tend to take things far too personally.

> *The instinct of a man is to pursue everything that flies from him,*
> *and to fly from all that pursue him.*
> —*VOLTAIRE, FRENCH AUTHOR AND PHILOSOPHER*

One can see how Voltaire might have reached this conclusion, but like most of us he had yet to experience an unconditionally loving relationship. We are forced to play games with each other because most of us are not honest with ourselves and others about our needs. Most of us are living in fear of being hurt. To love unconditionally opens us up to feeling vulnerable and to feeling pain. But if we enter into a relationship from a place of openness, clarity, and mutual understanding, it's less likely that assumptions will take over. Assumptions are based on fear, are rarely the truth, and are a catalyst for emotional pain.

One could argue that if one partner in a relationship feels the desire to seek physical relations outside the relationship, they are merely following their instincts. But if we can honestly look at the energy that is creating these desires, we can overcome them—should we wish to—sometimes quite easily. That voice pushing you to look outside your present relationship is the voice of the Ego, which doesn't want you to be happy. It thrives on separateness and will do anything to convince you to look elsewhere for love. Following the Ego, you break up with your partner or move away from what you already have—or even what you are about to or could have! If you find yourself doing this, do the puppet exercise from Chapter 12! If you can truly love and be loved, your desire to appease the Ego by going outside your relationship for satisfaction may just fall away.

Bear with me here, because this may seem counterintuitive, but you will find that if you *allow for the possibility* of distractions luring your lover away from you and truly understand the process that creates this distraction, your partner will feel more space and be less likely to venture there. If you make it clear that you are not imposing restrictions on your relationship, but allowing each person to experience freedom to choose, the mind will be less inclined to attempt its escape from perceived limitations.

Western culture tries to entice us away from anything we currently have toward whatever the advertiser wishes us to believe. A former clothing designer said it was his job to make women feel a) that they were ugly and miserable, and b) that his clothing could change that. We are constantly bombarded with advertising telling us our lives will be better with X, because X is now bigger, better, stronger, cleaner, and even smoother than it used to be—which of course means that we'll be more beautiful when we use it. We are taught that the grass is always greener over there, and that is easy to believe because we perceive that it isn't green where we currently stand.

This also blends into our relationships. Looking elsewhere will often be less fulfilling than you might expect. Dealing with what you have or who you are with right now will better your life from the inside out; it will draw more meaningful situations and higher-minded people into your new reality. But don't use someone solely for your own growth purposes unless you and that individual understand and have agreed that is your goal. You're going to encounter the same resistance and lessons you need to learn with this partner that you will with another, so why not do it with someone with whom you envision a long-term relationship? Assuming, of course, that is your goal.

NOTE: *Commit to going deeper; make it an intention that you renew each day and watch what happens!*

Another way through this perceived dilemma is truly committing to your beloved. If you both agree that most of your romantic relations have been missing a certain something, or that you were too easily frustrated by the other person's shortcomings, you can challenge yourselves to create a deeper level of loving. With presence, honesty, communication, and awareness, just about anything can be overcome. You will soon see that what you used to think of as faults will now be lovable quirks that make each person unique. You may even be less bothered that your beloved puts orange juice in his breakfast cereal!

Of course, if you both agree it is time to move on, bid adieu with love and with gratitude if possible. You'll grieve, of course, but that is okay and to be expected. You will have grown all you can within this relationship and, in time, will be ready for another.

The world is a looking glass and gives back to everyman the reflection of his own face.
—*WILLIAM MAKEPEACE THACKERAY, AUTHOR*

Unconditionally loving relationships are filled with acceptance and understanding. In this type of relationship, no one gets mad *at* their partner because they realize that getting angry is a reflection of their own self. If Mary gets mad at Tom for not cleaning up the kitchen, often the issue is about control, not just the dirty dishes.

No one can make you feel anything. If you believe a lover is seeking pleasure and contentment elsewhere, trust may be your issue. If you are being lied to and get upset, it is because in some way, honesty is your issue. All of these seemingly distressful situations are opportunities to heal.

Everything that irritates us about others can lead us
to an understanding of ourselves.
—*CARL JUNG, PSYCHIATRIST*

There's No Such Thing as a Victim of Circumstance

If you feel that it is always the "other guy" who is at fault, you have been misled. Notice, instead, the common element when you find the same thing keeps on happening to you— perhaps, for example, meeting several people who don't respect you. The common element is you. If you have an issue that began in childhood, or even an alternate existence, you will be sent as many opportunities necessary to heal that issue as you need. The Universe supports your spiritual growth, no matter what. The people it sends are always a gift.

When she didn't return his phone calls, it was an opportunity to forgive a per-
ceived lack of integrity. Apparently, he didn't do too well because, after they broke
up, he met quite a few people who did not return phone calls, either. Finally, he
saw how he was attracting more of the same! It was time to use the Five Steps!

If you are continually meeting people with whom you share a romantic interest and the relationship only goes so far, and it happens again and again, the Universe is telling you that you have an issue about getting close to someone. To experience a close romantic relationship, it will be necessary for you to open your heart. When you do so, you will attract another person in a similar state. They will see that you are open to love and will be more inclined to be open as well. If you have been open to learning from each of these experiences, you will notice that in your romantic history, each person you have met was more open than the previous partner. If you have not been learning from these relationships, you will have drawn to you the same type of person over and over (same boyfriend, different face), creating an unending list of opportunities to heal.

The person who drops you off at the airport in one city is
the same person who picks you up in the next.
—*MICHAEL RYCE, ND*

Frustration

Even if we are practicing awareness, there may be moments when something we are attempting to create—a relationship, abundance, health—will not manifest the way we wish it to, or even at all. At that point, you may get upset and frustrated.

We have been living a particular way for quite a while, and as a result it may take some time to integrate this new thought process. Don't get down on yourself: falling short is often what helps us grow. Recognize that you fell off the horse, and jump back on. You cannot learn to ride a horse by reading about it in a book; you have to actually ride one. When frustration occurs, it is time to step back and look at the concept of frustration—notice it only occurs when things don't go the way we *think* they should. Again, this is a great example of human arrogance. Thinking we always know the best way to do anything is the surest way to prevent learning anything new and can be a block to creating the life you desire. If you are too full to swallow your pride, it might be time to diet.

O, Wherefore Art Thou, Soul Mate?

If you believe in soul mates, then have fun with that concept. No one is trying to change your mind. However, if you invite the following definition of "soul mate" into your life, you will quickly see how it can relieve pressure and expectations about another person and improve your relationship with them and everyone you meet.

Ready?

YOU are your own soul mate. And so is EVERYONE else. Why not treat everyone you meet as special? Especially yourself! You may not wish to express love in the same way with all people, but you can love each one in your own unique way. If you're with the person you need to be with, you'll know it. They may be your soul mate, and a soul mate can last a day or a lifetime. Stay open to possibilities. Say yes to love.

NOTE: *That which came in with you is that with which you will exit. Befriend your own soul and the perfect things, people, and relationships will effortlessly come to you.*

CHAPTER 16

Perspective is Everything

When I was a boy of fourteen, my father was so ignorant
I could hardly stand to have the old man around.
But when I got to be twenty-one, I was astonished
at how much the old man had learned in seven years.

—*MARK TWAIN*

There will be as many perspectives as there are people for any particular event; each person will see that event in their own way. No view is intrinsically wrong, but some perspectives are healthy and others aren't. Which will you choose?

Bill decides that the driver who cut him off is wrong and will want revenge. His body tenses up, minimizing healthy blood flow to the muscles. Later on, he'll wonder why he is having neck pain. He was taught that "an eye for an eye" is a good thing, but is already too blind to see. It is likely that his blood pressure will be higher than that of others, and he may be at risk for coronary disease.

This is the "Type A" personality you so often hear about. He will be high-strung, tense, and anxious. He will seek revenge on people who do not even wish him harm. He will see the negative in people no matter what the situation is, and be the aggressor out of fear of being a victim. In his mind, he must get what he can whenever he can—at any cost. "Type A" people may get some things they desire in the short term, but this mindset will be damaging in the long term.

The mind is its own place, and in itself can create a heaven
out of hell or a hell out of heaven.

—*JOHN MILTON, AUTHOR, FROM "PARADISE LOST"*

In contrast, Wendy will think, "Okay, the person who cut me off was in a hurry, and I am not. I am still whole, my car has not been damaged, and I am no worse off than

I was a few moments ago." Wendy is even-tempered, calm, and more understanding of her choices. She not only lets things roll off her but she is a mirror that repels negative energy. She understands that she has choice in the present moment, and can safely surrender to situations that cannot be controlled. She has conditioned herself to make rational decisions based on the circumstances of each moment. People will want to be with her because she sees and recognizes the beauty in everyone, even before they see it themselves. She knows that how she sees someone will affect her communication with that person. She is open and nonjudgmental, creating space for others to be open as well. All of this doesn't mean that she is blind to truth; however, it does mean that she can stay clear of Bill, or deal with him well enough not to take on any of his negative energy. She releases fear and allows love into and from her heart. Her behavior is described in the Indian concept of *Namaste*.

> *In India, when we meet and part we often say, "Namaste,"*
> *which means I honor the place in you where the entire universe*
> *resides. I honor the place in you of love, of light, of truth, of peace.*
> *I honor the place within you where, if you are in that place in you,*
> *and I am in that place in me, there is only one of us.*
> —*UNKNOWN AUTHOR*

Everything is Temporary

NOTE: *Holding too fervently onto your past can prevent you from living in bliss, and yet the past is the very stairway that can bring you there.*

All thoughts and fears, loves and flings, and hopes and dreams are temporary. That job you think you'll be in for the rest of your life—temporary. The car you just spent way too much money on is temporary. Your marriage till death do you part—yes, it's temporary, too. You as a physical entity are temporary. Though your spirit never dies, your body changes every second. New cells are constantly replacing older cells. The pain in your neck? Temporary. The tumor in your lung? Yes, you guessed it, it's temporary. As soon as you've experienced it, the tumor will never exist the same way. That moment is gone. The past is dust. And every seven years, you are entirely new. Is this comforting or scary?

> *Body as process: Your skin cells are replaced once a month, liver every*
> *six weeks, skeleton every three months, DNA every six weeks.*
> —*DR. DEEPAK CHOPRA*

Try to embrace each yoga posture as if it is a one-of-a-kind. Even though you may have performed that asana hundreds of times before, it's different each time! Your entire life is like this—temporary. One day you are here, the next you are not. If you are working toward releasing attachments, this could be quite freeing. Think about the fact that nothing is permanent. Do you feel lighter, perhaps? By knowing that all things will pass, you can better release attachments to the past and fears of the future.

> *If everything is an illusion and nothing exists,*
> *I definitely overpaid for my carpet.*
> —*WOODY ALLEN, COMEDIAN AND FILM DIRECTOR*

Any concept will ultimately disappear upon analysis, and that is because, ultimately, everything we think we can see is an illusion. If there were only one reality, changing our perspective would change nothing. While any talk of illusionary realities may not seem relative to you who may be looking for a way out of a situation or a way to reduce some symptoms, I invite you to drop deeper into the rabbit hole. Of course, what we see is real—on the **macro**cosm. What we're inviting you now to do is live from the **micro**cosm. Living from here lets you see the illusion of physical reality clearer. Living from here is what spurs the most profound miracles to happen. To the spirit world, no miracles or healings are more or less important, bigger or smaller, better or worse—they just are. Because of this, one's energy is best put toward more gratitude and happiness than awe—thinking like Spirit does.

> *If everything is an illusion,*
> *why not pick one that works for you?*
> —*JAYADEV, YOGA INSTRUCTOR*

Living in awareness that everything is energy that is manipulated by thought, we can create what we wish to experience in less time than ever before. When living life AWARE of this fact, everything changes. The first few minutes of the day set the tone for the entire day. So begin with this simple exercise rather than throwing your alarm clock against the wall:

Each morning, write down your intention for the day. It can be as simple as "Today, I wish to embody compassion in all things that I do and toward all people whom I encounter." Make it a "to-do and to-be" list as opposed to the typical "to-do" list, and watch what happens! Examples: I will wash the dishes mindfully. I will attend the business meeting with a more open mind. I will call my parents because I want to do so, not because I have to.

Detoxification and Natural "Side Effects"

*We have to ask ourselves whether medicine is to remain a humanitarian
and respected profession, or a new but depersonalized science
in the service of prolonging life rather than diminishing human suffering.*
—ELISABETH KÜBLER-ROSS, PSYCHIATRIST,
AUTHOR OF "ON DEATH AND DYING"

In some cases, people may feel worse before feeling better. In traditional science this is often called a healing crisis; in more New Age thinking it is seen as a healthy detoxification. Years of internal grief or anger are rising to the surface for healing and, initially, can produce what is considered sickness, lethargy, or exacerbation of physical and/or emotional symptoms. This is the manifestation of resistance, for if we were truly open, these feelings would surface and release rather quickly. Few of us can be that open, so it's best to just recognize and accept that lack of openness for what it is, then work through the resistance. I think that most people would be willing to feel miserable for even a few days if they knew their spiritual DNA was being rebooted toward a higher vibration and better long-term health!

Our current healthcare system has convinced us that we need to stop any discomfort at once with medications. From a runny nose to serious pain, and everything in between, physical discomfort is seen as a horrible thing; yet, it's totally normal. Most medications cover up the energy at the causal level, leading more pain and illness to come out, sometimes years later. More alternative healthcare modalities recognize this and teach clients to stay present and breathe through it, for true healing lies just on the other side of discomfort.

Christine is having a difficult time with headaches. After asking the appropriate questions, we realize she is harboring intense anger at her mom. The headaches began shortly after her mom was diagnosed with lung cancer and given one year to live. Her mom created the conditions to manifest lung cancer by smoking cigarettes heavily for many years and repressing her emotions. We discuss how having anger toward her mom is not beneficial to anyone involved. Granted it is a normal reaction, but at this point, the anger isn't helping. Assuming her mom wants to recover, how will her daughter's anger help her or her daughter? Assuming she does not want to recover, what good will her daughter's anger provide? In less than twenty minutes, Christine says she's been selfish and has already started to release some of the rage. Her headache is dramatically lessened.

We say *assuming her mom wants to recover* or *assuming she does not want to recover* as a reminder to understand and accept that her mom's soul has a higher agenda than we are consciously aware of. Christine may miss her mom, and, yes, even be mad at her for leaving, but they will see each other again in whatever form that may be; that much is certain.

Why should I fear death? If I am, death is not. If death is, I am not.
Why should I fear that which cannot exist when I do?
—EPICURUS, PHILOSOPHER

CHAPTER 17

Seeing the Bigger Picture

NOTE: *Any activity done to anyone at anytime against his or her will without full knowledge of both the details of the event and its possible consequences is best dealt with quickly and efficiently so that this type of injustice is learned from and, therefore, prevented from reoccurring. The question here is: "What is meant by dealt with?"*

In mid-2002, and again in 2010, there was a media blitz reporting on priests who had sexually molested young males. The emphasis by the media and especially those within the religion itself was on revenge, punishment, and getting rid of the perpetrators. This made sense because their own religion told them that God would act with these same energies, too. However, from a more empowering understanding, no inquiry took place that sought to understand why it had happened in the first place. Wouldn't determining this missing piece of the puzzle help it from reoccurring and remove the weed at its root?

The perpetrator knows that what he did was wrong, although at the moment of infraction he apparently justified it. He already knows that to do anything to another without their consent is improper. He already knows that to do anything to a minor who does not fully understand the action or the consequences of that act is reprehensible. So, knowing all of this, why did he do it?

There were all kinds of laws being presented on how to deal with these men, and not a single one of them even began to look at a possible cause of these actions. There were proposals of zero-tolerance that included banning the perpetrator from any church, even if their injurious acts occurred several decades earlier. Please be clear, we are not condoning this activity in any way, but emphasis on the punishment will not make the problem go away. There was something all these men had in common to have justified doing—and in some cases repeating—this violent, unloving act that went against everything they'd ever been taught. And that is where the problem lies—in everything they'd ever been taught.

*Answer me and take your time, what could be the awful crime he could do
at so young an age?... All these cold and rude things that you do I
suppose you do because he belongs to you. And instead of love...
you've given him these cuts and sores that don't heal with time or with age.*
—*NATALIE MERCHANT /ROBERT BUCK, SINGER/SONGWRITERS,*
"WHAT'S THE MATTER HERE?"

Any person or group of people when told what to do and what not to do, will eventually rebel. It is the nature of the soul to express joyous, boundless freedom; inhibiting it in any way will create the energy of rebellion. Our freedom of choice was limited before we even knew it existed, and we will remain a victim of everyone else's perception of reality until we consciously commit to begin doing otherwise. This is why adults describe their child as going through their "Terrible Twos" when describing a toddler's minor attempts at independence. But what can a child at that age do to warrant such a malevolent nickname for their most tender years? It is when a child begins to say "no" that this energy is seen, but instead of it being recognized for what it is, as a soul just wishing to express its freedom and explore on its own, parents and caretakers get into a power struggle with a two-year-old! They will yell, take away food, distract, or even strike the child in this most lopsided and ridiculous of power struggles. The parent or caretaker who does this feels it is normal if he or she was brought up in that way and never questioned that pattern. You will note that anyone who tries to control another person (or even an animal) is literally fighting their own issue with the exact same energy that created it.

If a child is crabby, put them in water.
—*SARK, AUTHOR*

When this inhibiting behavior is continued, children will eventually rebel against what seems like everyone and everything. As they get older, they will try to tell you what they are feeling if you let them. If you are so hung up on dictating what you think is best for the child, you will not hear them, nor will they feel safe to discuss it. They will then do things to assert their individuality that seem ridiculous to you. Be it body piercing, drinking, or just being angry at you and everyone and everything, it is only because they are tired of being told what to do and what not to do. You are raising them the same way you were raised, and do not see what is really happening clearly enough to make a change. In extreme cases, teenagers can become angry, ill-tempered, or even abusive. This does not mean your child is bad, and it does not mean you are a bad parent. *It is solely the child trying to live, experience, and learn on their own, and you have yet to accept that fact.* It is perfectly natural to want for them what you feel is best, but when that is dictated as opposed to being discussed, problems will arise that could have been avoided if you knew the cause (in this case, the desire of the soul) beforehand.

How does this relate to the priests?

Telling a teenager whose hormones are going wild not to use his or her urges is often devastating to their full expression of sexuality, leading to difficulty with intimacy, too. Societies that embrace their sexuality will always have fewer incidences of sex-related crimes and disease, which are the end results of repression, anger, and control issues. When religion tells you not to practice sexual relations until you are married, it not only puts enormous pressure on the marriage but inhibits the body's normal urges and convinces you that they are wrong. Remember, *wrong* is a made-up term for what you do not agree with, or in this case, what the Church would have you agree with.

New definition of **Arrogance** \ 'ar-ʃ-gʃn(t)s \ **n**: to presume you know more than love does.

The Creator would never give something to you, then demand that you not use it. This is the personification of God that religions have used to keep you in place; and an entire theology of guilt, shame, painful childbirths, "illegitimate" children, and STD's were born around it. How could a being that is everything, has everything, and knows everything ever have any desires that could be unfulfilled? How could this being have any needs for itself that can go unmet? For some people, it is difficult to imagine a God without needs because we are seemingly filled with so many.

Many of these accused priests (as well as many others) were brought up and conditioned to deny their natural urges. Homosexuality is merely a sexual preference, not a disease, and is certainly not a sin in the eyes of God. In fact, no sexual relations between consenting adults is sinful. The priests were taught that homosexuality is a sin, so they repressed their natural urges. However, like the rain clouds that consistently fill with drops of water, everything eventually has its breaking point. Unfortunately, the priests' actions targeted innocent children, probably because there was less of a chance of getting caught if they could convince the child not to say anything.

> NOTE: *The perpetrators are victims themselves of a code of ethics gone horribly awry from true human nature; the unnatural mandate to curb very natural physical desires.*

Perhaps they went into the priesthood thinking it was a way to get closer to God—looking for understanding or forgiveness for what they'd been taught was wrong. Perhaps they sought the priesthood thinking abstinence would cleanse them of those thoughts that they believed would offend God. Yet, how could a being that has already seen everything and never judged anything ever be offended by this behavior? Perhaps these priests were molested themselves as children? They had to learn about boundaries, or lack thereof, from somewhere. It's time to stop the insanity!

It is impossible to cure anything with the same mind that created it.
—ALBERT EINSTEIN, PHYSICIST

We've all been programmed to avenge a wrongdoing, but similar to treating a symptom rather than a cause, throwing the guilty behind bars without some sort of understanding of why it occurred in the first place doesn't heal. First off, how can a randomly selected jury, all at different levels of spiritual understanding, judge anyone else? Who are we to think we can judge anyone? Can we even begin to do so without knowing the bigger picture? After death, Source tells me, souls get a chance to review their past, and we choose what's next. So, what comes around does go around, but it's by choice of the individual. Second, calling a prison a "correctional facility" is a euphemism. You might as well take away people's civil liberties and make up some crazy euphemism like The Patriot Act! *Indeed, the typical legal system and its oft-subsequent imprisonment—without true correction done at a soul level with awareness and right action—will reinforce the lack of love within the person that created the incorrect perception to begin with, further cementing the underlying repressed emotions.* And we wonder why we have repeat offenders!

There may be some priests who are about to engage in this behavior and are now pondering if the punishment is worth the act. But if the urges are too strong, the fear of punishment is of no use. Anything is possible in a fit of rage, which is merely the end result of repressed anger or, in this case, repressed sexuality. Rage can cloud our ability to reason to such an extent that individuals have planned and committed murder, and never once did the fear of punishment—whether life imprisonment or the death penalty—stop them.

NOTE: *See the bigger picture in everything, and your life will change dramatically. That is of course, unless you like things the way they are.*

Violence

Revenge, hostility, and war are part of our culture (ultimately, because we live in a world where we learn about anything in relation to its opposite). But these violent tendencies can be minimized, even eliminated, if we look at the bigger picture, accept it, understand it, and act upon it. We can learn from the past and not feel doomed to repeat it. What we've been doing hasn't worked yet, and it will continue to not work until a change is made.

The United Nations has a tendency to believe that the best way to deal with unco-operative nations is to impose sanctions. But knowing what we know about the nature of the soul, both individual and collective, we have to ask: what happens when more restrictions are placed upon millions of people because their government doesn't want to agree to something? Those people eventually will rebel, and then their own government may take action on them, and rarely does diplomacy play any part in it. But diplomacy is the only thing that can create lasting peace. Consider our current challenges with terror-ism. Terrorism is a radical ideological approach to changing things that attracts followers caught up in its message. We can root out, try, and condemn terrorists all we like, but ideas cannot be erased so easily. As more alleged terrorists are killed, their cause can actu-ally gain momentum. Friends and family members of those killed now have a new enemy that they may not have had before.

Everyone wants something. Diplomacy is an effective means to determine what those wants are, and then for others to act accordingly. We're all in this together and we can only escape the pain and suffering by working together.

More traditional minds are convinced that things were better years ago before com-puters, instant messaging, cell phones, and media portrayals of violence as not only a normal occurrence but an effective way of dealing with a problem. The media was born out of our way of life; it is merely a much larger reflection of what has and already is oc-curring.

Those who wage war in the name of religion have failed to look beyond their religion to the faiths they oppose. If they did, they would recognize the same needs and desires they have—the same dreams, and fears, and the same loves.
—*THE DALAI LAMA*

Wars have been around forever. Anti-gun advocates claim it is the proliferation of guns that is the cause. This is assuming there was no violence in man before guns were invent-ed. Before guns, there were bows and arrows, before that there were spears, and before that there were clubs. Throughout much of the past, there have been poisons and torture and repressed sexuality. There have always been inferiority complexes cleverly disguised as superiority complexes (Ego) to the point of intolerance toward anyone who is seemingly different. All too often we have tried to convert people to a particular religion to "save" them, but if they refused to be saved, they were killed. Anyone who is seemingly different has been criticized, abused, locked away, or systematically murdered. The process has been given so many euphemisms—most act in the name of their God, whom they believe has chosen them as the greatest people to ever live and, therefore, has blessed them with this right.

Contradictions both condoning and condemning anything are abundant in many of the world's spiritual texts. One of the Ten Commandments instructs us not to commit adultery. That theme is constantly revisited in the Bible. Another says not to murder, yet the Bible is filled with people murdering one another. Even God, it is written, has killed out of anger. Why would God command, "Thou shalt not kill," and then smite one of his creations as is often written in the Bible? Assuming this all-loving being wanted someone dead, why would he be so lazy as to command a person or a group of people to do it for him? How can anything but more confusion arise from a book of such drastic contradictions?

Worse yet, we're taught never to question these written and rewritten words. An example of this rewording is the laws of mandated celibacy for priests in A.D. 1139, after more than 11 centuries of debate. With no heirs, all of a priest's inheritance would have to go to the Church! How convenient. But because it is written in the Bible, questioning is considered blasphemy. It is a system perfectly designed for self-perpetuation written by Ego-driven humans to satisfy their own desires.

Arguably the greatest playwright in the English language, William Shakespeare wrote plays about revenge, infidelity, and murder (the latter are euphemistically called romantic tragedies). Is this just beautiful prose, or are our collective selves being subjected to the scrutiny of a magnifying glass? Was Shakespeare really advocating murder as the ultimate revenge—a drastic method of dealing with normal emotions gone horribly astray? Or was he showing us at our worst, so that we could work to avoid it?

Oh No, You Didn't!

One of Shakespeare's most misunderstood themes is infidelity. This book advocates not putting down marriage itself, but to look at its present construction and figure out why it is not working; marriage as it is currently set up is actually creating what is called infidelity.

It is said that a marriage contract is a watered down version of a slavery contract. Indeed, with the promises of "love, honor, and OBEY" written right into the traditional wedding vows, that much is obvious. Such a promise in and of itself is a fallacy. How can anyone say what they definitely will do or be at any time in the future? Arrogance leads us to believe we can control the future, and that's just not possible.

Soul Desire

Human beings have countless desires (not just sexual ones), and to expect one person to fulfill them all is generally asking a lot. The only crime being committed is the restriction on the soul's urge to grow. Sometimes that is manifested in outrageous ways. We feel trapped by our spouse, and we think it is their fault. We think it is a sexually related issue, only to find out that after we engage in infidelity we are still left with the same emotional void that made us do it in the first place. Still being unfulfilled, we do it again, and not always with the same person! Eventually there is guilt, falling out of love, revenge, anger, and a spot on the Jerry Springer show.

All of this—including priests' molestation of minors—can be avoided if those involved make an effort to understand what is going on before things get out of hand. It is important to understand the nature of the soul and work with it, not against it.

Reread these passages when faced with your own challenges and, as time goes on, you'll be more able to think before you react. Know your truth and how to use it; act more lovingly and compassionately. This process alone can cause a chain reaction because others will notice your peace of mind, maybe even praise it, and wish to be near you. You will embody the change they've been waiting to see was possible. Let's change the judicial system to one of compassion and correction rather than revenge. And let's reduce the need for such a harsh judicial system by educating others about the soul's desires versus those of the Ego.

The Law of Resonance

How far you go in life depends on your being tender with the young,
compassionate with the aged, sympathetic with the striving
and tolerant of the weak and strong,
because someday in life you will have been all of these.
—*GEORGE WASHINGTON CARVER, EDUCATOR,*
AGRICULTURAL AND FOOD SCIENTIST, FARMER

The Law of Resonance states that whenever you commit to something new or have a spiritual shift, you will be sent persons and situations that embody the opposite energy shortly thereafter. For example, if you commit to being an honest person after years of lying, you will be sent dishonest people within a short period of time. Or if you've just committed to financial abundance, you may be asked for money on the street a bit more that day. Why does this sort of thing happen?

After we commit to something greater than our prior self, many become judgmental toward those who are still living where we've just come from. If Jerry's just quit smoking, even while knowing how difficult quitting can be, he often thinks less of Tony who is smoking near his office. Jerry will think or even tell Tony that he is weak-willed. He might even ask Tony to blow the smoke in another direction because the smell now makes him sick.

Jerry can also take a road less traveled. With love and understanding, Jerry can say, "Hey Tony, it was tough, but if I can quit, anyone can. I'm here for you if you need it." It is an opportunity, a gift. It's a chance to exercise compassion and love unconditionally, knowing that Tony is really a spiritual messenger reminding Jerry of what he used to be like! Jerry can now thank him and embrace his own past, knowing that he's raised his vibration. Through compassion and gratitude, Jerry will more likely continue to be smoke-free because what is sent out—in this case, support—is returned to the sender.

No two persons ever read the same book.
—EDMUND WILSON, CRITIC

It's time to practice tolerance and love for yourself and those you know. Start a support group. Give this book to a friend. Meditate. Love thy neighbor and thyself. For God's sake (literally, because you and God are one) do something! Be -cause of the wonderful things you do!

CHAPTER 18

A New and Overdue Perspective on Nutrition

In California, kindergarten children receive a coloring book from the California Milk Producers' Association. On the first page is an illustration of a man's face with the following text: "What did Dad eat today? If Dad has had his butter, Dad is happy. Draw a smile on his face. If Dad has not had his butter, Dad is sad." Then it says "If Dad has had his cheese today" and so on. You end up with one of two Dads: The one with the high-fat diet looks happy and healthy, and you can guess the rest. What's traditionally seen as a public service is really free advertising aimed at a vulnerable and captive audience.

—*JOHN ROBBINS, FROM "DIET FOR A NEW AMERICA"*

There are countless studies about nutrition and its effects on health and illness, and the results are often contradictory. Remember the Four Food Groups? It worked for a while—until it no longer did. How about the Food Pyramid? That, too, worked for a while—until it no longer did! In the last few years, numerous studies have concluded that in order to be healthy, one must maximize proteins; carbs have been declared the enemy. Yet others seem to feel that carbohydrates give people energy—many athletes "carbo-load" before a major event. Still others concluded that nutrition should be based on blood type. The only thing happening here is that most of us—even unconsciously—find evidence to support our version of reality.

Life is simple to a simple mind,
and complex to a complex mind.
—*MICHAEL RYCE, ND*

Wouldn't it be great to know what's good for you as an individual, and not what another person, study, or corporation says is good for you? How can we ever really know? You're about to find out.

If you're still with me, I congratulate you on your openness. But that's about to get tested again. Some of us have had experience using a pendulum, or dowsing, but not everyone understands why or how it works. Though I've heard many possibilities, and they're all fine if it works for you, not all of them work for everyone all of the time; this one does.

To utilize a pendulum for determining which foods strengthen or weaken you, let's note that energy leaves you and all things and goes outward in all directions. Each one of these things or people sends out energy at a particular frequency, and that frequency can be measured. But who wants to rely on expensive, high-tech machinery to measure a vibrational frequency? For less than a dollar, you can measure the energetic frequency of your prospective dinner!

Begin by making a pendulum out of dental floss and a paper clip, though I've found a cotter pin is a bit more successful. More helpful and life-changing information that costs less than a stick of gum? Yes! What did you expect? A shameless plug for my own line of highly receptive, energetic, calculating, dolphin-safe, oscillatory, organic, low-emission, quantum pendulums made of hemp in various chakra- based colors blessed by a rabbi?

Cut about 8 inches, or 20 centimeters of floss, and tie one end around the cotter pin's loop and you're done. You've just made your own pendulum. Hold your new energy-testing device by the non-cotter pin side as motionless as possible. Dangle it so that the cotter pin is a few inches over the food in question. After about 10 seconds, the cotter pin will begin moving. It is irrelevant if it is moving forward or backward, side to side, or dances in a circle; the fact is that the pendulum is "testing" the energetic frequency emanating from the food and showing you that it is vibrant. In just 10 seconds, you'll be able to see how much more vibrant an organic orange is when compared to any typical snack food. Foods that vibrate at a high frequency will cause the pendulum to move at a faster rate than those foods that are lifeless, and if food is a source of energy, which would you prefer to ingest?

If peanuts test as a good source of energy, you may feel you can eat them based on this test—not so, because you've only done the first part of the test—seeing what foods emanate a higher amount of energy. What if you are allergic to peanuts? Is there a way to determine not only what are good sources of high-energy food but also to test if that particular food is good for any particular person?

Yes, there is! Holism means to account for each person as a whole individual life force. We need to determine how to test each food energetically for each person.

Between all things that appear to be matter is an energetic matrix. As you move farther away from your prospective dinner, the strength of the matrix between you and it is decreased. That is why we test using the pendulum very close to the food in question. Likewise, you, too, emit energy at a particular frequency.

Halfway between the food in question and you, a new unit of energy is formed; we will call this energy unit the *fulcrum*. This fulcrum is the pivotal point between health and illness, energy or lethargy, and health or disease, when testing for individualized nutrition.

Hold the pendulum at the fulcrum for about 10 seconds. At that time, the pendulum will move a lot, a little, somewhere in between those two, or not at all. The amount that it moves is relative to the vibration of the energetic matrix that is formed at the fulcrum, and tells you what foods strengthen or weaken you on an individualized, or holistic, basis. Lots of movement? Enjoy. Little or none? Check, please. It's that simple. If you don't have a pendulum nearby, or don't want to use it at The Russian Tea Room, it's good to know that a little bit of anything probably will not hurt you (*sans* those things to which you believe you are allergic) in the way of overall health, weight gain, energy levels, etc., but too much of anything just might.

You will notice that those who do everything in moderation will generally be among the healthiest. Those pale and underweight people in health food stores are unhealthy not because of the bland "health food" but because of their excessive worry about eating healthily! Why is this so? Because (excluding rotten food, poisons, and so on) your state of mind while ingesting anything is often more important than the food itself!

Some monks actually count their chews to be more mindful; this slows down eating and relaxes the digestion process! Typically, after we've ingested enough food to get the energy and nutrients we need, many of us keep on eating because our awareness of satiety is dulled by watching television, conversation, reading, and the like. Eating more slowly and more mindfully will allow your body to get what it needs without the unbutton-the-pants-after-Thanksgiving-day-turkey feeling. You'll eat less, have more energy, and stay at a healthy weight. You'll even save money. Aren't you glad you're reading this?

Thoughts on Vegetarianism

Thought: Why does man kill? He kills for food.
And not only for food: frequently there must be a beverage.
—*WOODY ALLEN, AUTHOR*

For those who have chosen to be vegetarians, if your body responds better to this type of diet, then so be it. Aside from the seemingly equal number of both *warnings against* and *recommendations for* the nutritional aspects of vegetarianism, there is the energy factor to take into account.

According to any high-school science book, the amount of energy is decreased dramatically from layer to layer. That is to say, energy comes from the sun, is absorbed and used by vegetation, which is eaten by an animal—a cow, for example—whose muscles are then eaten by you. Yes, what you call meat is most often an animal's muscles—not something the meat and dairy associations announce to your five-year old in kindergarten. And in each layer of this transfer, up to 90 percent of the energy is lost as heat. Vegetarianism reduces one layer in the process; this provides more energy from the vegetables directly to you without the proverbial middle-cow.

Slaughterhouses and the farms where the animals are raised are often dismal places where animal cruelty is the norm. Cows are shot in the head after being pushed along in assembly line fashion, bulls are castrated without anesthesia, and pigs are altered in other violent and inhumane manners to render them more profitable for tomorrow's breakfast. Many are skinned or even cooked alive after living in cages no bigger than their bodies. They have no opportunity to exercise or any chance of freedom, and they are routinely injected with chemicals and hormones to maximize size, production, and thus profits. The close proximity causes fights among them and can lead to disease as animals are forced to live among (and eat) their own waste. All of this produces chemicals within the animal that are similar to that of our fight-or-flight response to stress. You are eating these fear-based chemicals among the awful diet of hormones and feces whenever you eat conventional chicken or a hamburger.

NOTE: *For more information on this, see* www.MeetYourMeat.Com. *For a G-rated version, see* www.TheMeatrix.com.

The greatness of a nation and its moral progress can
be judged by the way its animals are treated.
—MAHATMA GANDHI

When religions teach that harming your fellow humans to get your way is a God-given right, animal abuse and subsequent killing are seen as just another logical step in justified cruelty. The spiritual aspect, however, points out that humans have no right to abuse animals, much less each other. We order a hamburger and it doesn't look like a cow, but we are eating a cow's muscles. We order chicken cutlet and don't see the eyes, the feet, or the face, and happily ingest its muscles, too. If these animals were given a choice, do you think they'd choose to give up their life for you? Or, perhaps as some believe, they did choose that existence. Well, what do you think?

Plants have found a way to survive without killing;
maybe we're not as smart as we think we are.
—FRANCIS HALL, ACTOR

If you feel you cannot get by without animal products in your diet, use those labeled organic, or free-range, or pasture raised. These animals are fed better and are not given added hormones or other chemical injections. Also find out if the animals were raised humanely. The Certified Humane Raised and Handled program (as per their website) assures that in addition to the above, "animals are raised with shelter, resting areas, sufficient space and the ability to engage in natural behaviors." It may be a few dollars more, but the health benefits and the peace of mind in not supporting animal abuse will be well worth it.

> NOTE: *Eventually, you will pay—with your wallet or your health. Choose wisely.*

Either way, it's best to have and express reverence for all the foods you eat. Cultivate gratitude to the uncountable numbers of people involved in the system that brought you a banana from thousands of miles away that you can buy for a quarter on a street corner ($1 in a Manhattan deli). Should you eat an animal, express gratitude to its spirit. Smile at the cook in your favorite restaurant, and let her know she's made your day. Give your partner a hug and tell them you appreciate their cooking for you, or better yet, bless each ingredient as you prepare a dish for yourself and your partner, friend, or family. My grandmother and her husband made lasagna that no one could duplicate, even when the exact recipe was passed down to younger generations. Undoubtedly, their secret ingredient was their love for us, and the preparation and cooking over several days' time.

"No, Thanks, Not For Me." —The Mindset of Limitations

Why is it best not to limit yourself with labels of vegetarian, lacto-vegetarian, carnivore, and so on? Because the connotation around the label of vegetarianism is "*No* meat, *no* eggs, *no* fish, and so on," —this continual "no" sets up a mind-set of limitations. Better to concentrate on what you do eat!

When you deny an aspect of yourself with a negative mind-set, you are denying your wholeness. On a subconscious level, you desire wholeness, so you will crave whatever it is you are telling yourself not to have, eat, or be. When you get a little taste of it, you often binge. All dieters know about this. But if you allow yourself the occasional sweet, you will be less likely to crave a lot of it. Think of it like homeopathy; just a little dab will do ya!

By testing with the pendulum and not subjecting yourself to limitations, your body will slowly minimize and eventually eliminate all cravings for foods or drinks that are harmful to it! By using the pendulum, the best choice is given to us—easier than choosing between McDonalds or Burger King.

A quick side-note on these fast-food giants: Have you noticed they load their burgers with tons of "fixings?" This seems to be an effort to cover up, not enhance, the flavor of the meat. The meat itself has no flavor left. It is like eating cardboard. For those who still eat meat, I dare you to do a side-by-side comparison of how you feel when eating a fast-food chicken sandwich versus an organically produced version. Go on, try it. What are ya, chicken?

It's also interesting to note that some indigenous peoples ingest pure, unaltered dirt to obtain their minerals. While this may lack a bit of flavor for most of us, it seems to be not only logical but highly cost effective. People the world over have ingested what is considered unthinkable to others. What is considered appalling to some people may be the highest delicacy or best source of nutrition elsewhere. These "primitive" people often have less incidence of major disease than "civilized" societies.

NOTE: *Take into account what we now know about muscles; they are warehouses of emotions. With all the aforementioned abuse that animals are victim to, what exactly are you ingesting along with the meat itself?*

Pendulum Testing for Causes of Pain and Illness

The pendulum can also be used to determine if a chakra is open or closed. An open chakra is a sign of a healthy amount of energy—vitality, and thus health, can then be expected. A closed chakra needs to be opened to enjoy optimal living. Hold the pendulum in front of any chakra and within about 10 seconds, watch it dance—or not! If it dances, that person is open and vibrant. If it is stationary, you might want to call that bodyworker whose card you threw out last week.

If a particular chakra is closed, look up what emotions are held in that chakra and see if that finding resonates with something in your life. Once you have this new awareness, practice The Five Steps to Health (daily, if need be).

CHAPTER 19

"Addictions"

Healing with Source Example No. 4

"Laura" attended a lecture I gave in San Diego. She resonated with much of the information but wanted individualized attention and more clarification on what was causing her to remain overweight for much of her life, so she booked a private session the next day. When I created the safe space for her to feel her feelings and begin speaking about her past, she shared that she was molested much of her early teenage life by her dad. Her body was tense with anger and sadness from a childhood that seemed lost; it permeated her being.

I saw that her lack of ability to talk about this to anyone else caused a major blockage in her throat chakra, which then affected the energy going in and coming from her thyroid, affecting her metabolism. She had been diagnosed by Western medicine as having hypothyroidism, for which they recommended medication. Also, she'd dieted and exercised for years and years and was unable to shed the weight. When I told her what was happening—that she'd only been addressing two-thirds of the weight issue (exercise and diet, but not the emotional aspects)—she seemed to get it, and I didn't hear from her until a year later. In a seemingly random email, she reminded me who she was and about our session, and then added "Somehow I was able to get up the courage to speak with my molester. I was no longer that scared, little girl. I owned my power. And in the last year, 40 pounds have been shed almost effortlessly. The hypothyroidism is gone, and I feel great!"

Overeating and Obesity

Genetics are not the cause of obesity. Food itself does not cause obesity; whether it is labeled a fat, a carbohydrate, or a protein is irrelevant. Stagnant lifestyle alone does not cause obesity. Eating too much of almost *any* food to fill in the perceived missing parts of the self causes obesity.

Many people reach for food to assist in getting through what seems to be troubled times. Oral satisfaction is a one of the original control mechanisms, but now it is the adult who is covering up the symptoms in an attempt to control what seems to be out of control! Blaming genetics seems to be a way of understanding the problem, but that leaves the person with a victim consciousness—giving in to believing they are *destined* to be obese. This is *defeatist thinking* that will leave them obese. An article in *Time* magazine stated that all persons are born with genetic possibilities of every type, and that the conditioning, or learning process, turns these possibilities on or off. This means that nature and nurture both exist! We get to choose!

If there's no such thing as happiness,
we'll just have to be happy without it.
—UNKNOWN AUTHOR

Children pick up on everything that adults do. They learn that the instant gratification received from eating is a way of filling in their perceived inner voids. Parents will often project their unhappiness on their children, and feed them whenever they appear upset—in actuality, the child might merely be looking for attention. Parents don't see why their child is obese at three years old. If it's the parent's issue that is causing it, then *that* is what needs to be addressed.

To love oneself is the beginning of a lifelong romance.
—OSCAR WILDE, AUTHOR

Dieting doesn't work in the long term because it does not address the causal factors—in fact, it inhibits more than frees! When dieting does appear effective, it does so for only the short-term; most persons put the weight back on. By eating well, exercising regularly, and addressing the energetic and emotional bodies, you are making changes that will very likely become habit. You'll increase self esteem, feel healthier, and you'll be more fulfilled with less. This enjoyment of life reduces the body's NEED for instant gratification items like junk food, alcohol, or even sex. As *desire* replaces *need*, you will be much more attractive to people, in general, but especially to your partner or even potential partner. Your desire to ingest mind-numbing chemicals will be replaced with a zest for life that nothing outside the body can match. There will be no need to overdo anything because you will be satiated in less time—not because food doesn't taste good but simply because you've had enough of it.

Smoking

Cigarettes can provide instant gratification even though, when we smoke, we inhale as many as 4,000 chemicals per breath—including rat poison. People will say they enjoy smoking, when it is often the oral satisfaction combined with deep breaths that bring pleasure. How can nicotine, a known stimulant, assist in relaxing someone? It doesn't. What relaxes the smoker is the distraction away from the perceived stressor (the "cigarette break"), the numerous energy-reducing and mind-numbing chemicals, and mostly, breathing deeply! The latter sends messages of relaxation to your mind and body—this can be done without the rat poison. You don't see too many deep-breathing yogis lighting up outside the ashram!

Unfortunately, we've all been conditioned by the tobacco industry to feel we are powerless. Big Tobacco targets the Ego with its seductive advertising, seizing its attention, and we start believing the message more than our true selves. When the tobacco companies show us young, sexy models enjoying fun activities with other beautiful people—all with cigarettes in hand but none with yellow teeth—we believe that smoking can be fun. Their products ruin our smiles and skin. Advertisers mysteriously leave out the fog of smoke at the top of any bar scene, leading us to believe it is healthier than it really is. They purposely infuse their product with uncountable toxic chemicals including things shown to be addictive. Sure, the government forced them to place a warning on the box, yet the sale of these cancer sticks is still legal. As author Neale Donald Walsch so aptly put it: we have a paradigm where quick suicide is illegal, and slow suicide via cigarettes and alcohol is called commerce. Cigarettes are easily obtained by anyone—even minors. Tobacco executives have said under oath that their products do not have any correlation to disease. Selective vision drives them to the bank in their Mercedes Benz and we drive our beloved to the cemetery in a hearse.

A sticker on the dashboard of my junior high school bus:

CANCER CURES SMOKING

Violence, Control, and Drinking

Drinking alcohol will turn you into the same
$%@#$%@ your father was.
—GEORGE CARLIN, COMEDIAN

Violence has been around since the origin of our species—long before it began to be portrayed so ubiquitously on television and in movies, beginning in the 20th century. But many people are quick to blame anyone or anything but themselves for their behavior choices, and may not take the time to look closely and see that our media are creating fantasies; they do not show the real-life consequences of violence. Violence in the world of mass media is contained within a half-hour or hour-long show on television, or a two-hour movie, then the problem is gone because the good guy beat up the bad guy. But the real question is: how good is the "good guy" when he uses the tools of evil to defeat his enemy?

Those brought up amid household violence—a tool used by strong but insecure people to oppress the weak and powerless—often seek to fill the void with food and other substance abuse, but they will never succeed. Children sometimes get back at being controlled by re-creating and trying to work out their home situations elsewhere—but from the opposite perspective. An example would be if a child feels small and unimportant at home, he will project these behaviors onto a schoolteacher, attempting to make the schoolteacher feel small and unimportant. If this behavior is caught early enough in the classroom, it can be worked with before it becomes problematic. These behaviors are not inborn but learned; if a child is raised with love, he or she will love.

Drinking alcohol to excess is often blamed on genetics as well, but this does nothing to change the existing situation. If a child is raised in an environment of drinkers, they will get the message that drinking is a normal method of dealing with pain and filling in the perceived missing pieces of life. Of course, as in all situations of parental imprinting, free will does eventually play a part. Even if these messages are installed from a young age, ideally, as we grow, we'll see what works and what doesn't— given what we wish to accomplish—and act accordingly. Bottom line: If a child is raised with unconditional love, she will find it easier to love unconditionally. Draw that line here and now!

CHAPTER 20

HIV and AIDS

NOTE: *Time does not heal all; it only buries the hurt.*

After reading most of this book or experiencing a lecture or workshop on mind-body medicine, people will often ask about how to work with more serious diseases, such as HIV and AIDS. It is my belief, inspired by the small amount of volunteer energy work I have done with People With AIDS (PWAs) and then a whole lot of channeling about it, that a more serious illness like AIDS can also be addressed in the mind-body paradigm. We must consider its causes, and know that extended periods of time with unaddressed causes has allowed deeper states of illness to manifest. As a matter of policy; however, I never "treat" a "disease." But because I do get asked about, what to date has been called the worst of them all, AIDS, I will share these comments.

In the late 1970s and early 1980s, several groups of people began to contract a series of symptoms in alarming numbers. A few years later, a virus called HIV was discovered, which became known as the virus that causes AIDS. Intravenous drug users and male homosexuals seemed to constitute the greatest percentage of sufferers, and it was said that the virus was spread by bodily fluid exchange, such as that which occurs more often in the sharing of needles and anal intercourse. Though these are obvious factors, few understood the virus and its origin. Many people theorized about where it actually started—and all were examples of the soon-to-be discussed, "The Theory Decides What Can Be Observed."

As I explained at the beginning of this book, not all individuals who come into contact with a virus manifest it in their bodies. There is a reason for this—the strength of the immune system. No one ever bothered to figure out *why these particular groups of people* were more susceptible to being infected than others. *That* is what I call the X Factor.

Homosexual men, who, aside from their sexual identity, are no different from anyone else, are often highly oppressed because they are often viewed as different from a *so-called norm*. Many homosexuals are told by their religion that their God does not love them as they are! This is pounded into people's skulls, and it could not be farther from the truth! If Tim is a young male attending religious services and is force-fed this model, and one day he acknowledges that his sexual attraction is different from what he's been told is acceptable, *how would that affect Tim's health?* The same God that Tim grew up worshipping and revering as the All-Mighty and All-Forgiving, now—in his mind—hates him. If Tim buys into the idea that even God hates him, what energies will that create? How will he feel about himself?

Intravenous drug use is a temporary escape from emotional or physical pain and toward pleasure, usually engaged in by people with chronic low self-esteem. Would someone who truly loved themselves regularly inject poisons into their body? Most substance abusers have had difficult life circumstances, some filled with varied forms of abuse. Poor upbringings due to economic hardships, strewn lifestyles of family members, and a lack of spirituality based on faith (and not teachings) and more can also be involved. These are not bad people—they are in pain and do not have the appropriate tools for awareness or self-transformation. Send them compassion!

In both groups of people who were originally identified as the main carriers of HIV, the immune system has been compromised due to their separation from their essential being, often referred to as low self-esteem. That is the X factor! If religion didn't teach gay men that they are unloved by God, and those who use drugs were taught to love themselves enough not to inject, HIV might not have ever been an issue. But it is and we have to deal with it. If any of this has challenged your reality and made you think a bit—good for you! If you vehemently disagree—good for you, too!

Since its initial outbreak, many other people who weren't gay men or intravenous drug users have, unfortunately, been infected. Here is where collective and individual fears are engaged.

Repressed and prolonged fear reduces the efficiency of the immune system. Fear-based, self-fulfilling prophecies of becoming infected with any disease can actually steer the person in the direction where the possibilities of being infected are increased. All thoughts are creative! Once people live in fear, anything is possible. See the documentary, *Bowling for Columbine* by Michael Moore for more on how fear can permeate a society and lead to irrational, unloving acts.

Surely, AIDS has affected more than homosexuals and intravenous drug users. Source says that this transmission can be from any or all of the following:

- **Lack of:** quality medical care, nutrition, and condoms. Though obvious, susceptibility to even minor illness or disease is increased if these are not readily available.
- **Effective birth control** is rare. Many children are born out of necessity or lack of planning, and not out of desire to increase the amount of love in the world. When

a child perceives their very existence as a burden, their immune system will be weakened.

- **Fear.** In an environment of poverty, anger, political unrest, and lack of a stable group of family and community, fear reigns supreme and affects illness and disease creation and transmission.

- **Lack of love-based spirituality.** Some religions teach that some people are unworthy of love. Victim consciousness and lack of self-love and acceptance taught by religions actually reduce the immune system's efficiency.

I honor the people infected, the researchers, and the wonderful doctors hoping to find a cure. Unfortunately, good-intentioned people in modern medicine and science have spent vast time, effort, and money trying to suppress the symptoms, as though that equals a cure, without recognizing the underlying causes. This research, though a godsend for some, sometimes leaves more to be desired and could be expanded: We owe it to those infected and those at risk to research ALL possibilities! Let's change the mind-set of the typical walkathon and telethon toward educathon and preventathon!

> NOTE: *Viruses are created by the collective unconscious; by looking for an external force thought to be responsible for previously unknown symptoms. HIV was unconsciously created by humans; not as an all-powerful weapon by an enemy government, or by an angry God looking to punish, but merely as an end result of looking for it.*

If we looked at ourselves more from a larger point of view, and we understood the power of our thoughts, words, and actions, maybe we could teach our children self-love, openness, honesty, and respect in addition to reading, writing, and arithmetic. Isn't it time to recognize people for who they are and not label them according to sexual preference, color, or religion? Maybe acceptance and understanding is all it takes to live in better health, and ultimately, in peace.

CHAPTER 21

The Science of Mind-Body Medicine

There is no prescribed route to follow to arrive at a new idea.
You have to make the intuitive leap. But, the difference is
that once you've made the intuitive leap, you have to justify it
by filling in the intermediate steps.
—*DR. STEPHEN HAWKING, PHYSICIST*

Most people are only able to see what they wish to see, and hear only what they wish to hear. It takes great determination to let into our reality information that contradicts what we already believe, since those thoughts often get filtered out. Obviously, many people have difficulty acknowledging they could be mistaken, but the only way to learn something new is to welcome alternative viewpoints.

We must be like the best scientists, who put aside everything they've ever known to allow room for something new to be discovered—or created. After doing experiments in which light would, indeed, do what he predicted it would do, Albert Einstein stated, "The theory decides what can be observed." This sentence, in addition to being a simplification of quantum physics, explains the variety of diagnoses and treatments recommended by different practitioners for the same group of symptoms, as happened to me and countless others. The existing paradigms of these practitioners dictated their explanations and understandings of what they were seeing. Certainly, their paradigms of reality need to be respected and understood, but they are no less or more real than your own. You can choose to live in someone else's reality if it seems to fit, or, even better, start exercising the creative power within you and create your own.

*The Theory **Decides** What Can Be Observed* can also be written as *The Theory **Creates** What Can Be Observed*! Such is the power of the mind (consciously or unconsciously) that we create or draw to us everything that we have ever experienced, or wish to experience now and in the future. All of life is a manifestation of thought; when thought is combined it blends into the Unified Field of Consciousness and Energy, of which we all are a part, and creates larger forms of energy and information that can then be utilized more readily.

The Theory Deciding What Can Be Observed

It was a commonly held opinion based on medically proven facts in the 1970s that ulcers were caused by spicy foods, so people cut back on spicy foods. Apparently, this understanding had a negligible effect on the rate of ulcers because their incidence did not decrease. In the 1980s, this medically proven fact was seen as false evidence—new medical evidence concluded that ulcers were caused by stress. Knowing this, people tried to minimize stress. The rates of ulcers still did not decrease and, in the 1990s, even newer medical evidence concluded that ulcers were a result of a particular strain of bacteria. Each decade, reliable and repeatable scientific studies found contrasting results to studies conducted just a few years earlier. A good question is: "So, what causes ulcers?" But a much better question would be: "*Why* did each of these studies show different results?"

The persons responsible for the studies on ulcers had their own ideas and their own agenda. Though most likely an unconscious process, their thoughts created or drew to them exactly what they predicted or theorized they might see. By applying *The Theory Decides What Can Be Observed* to anything, you can see how each study showed something different while using even the most advanced scientific methods. Therefore, it can be said that even science is not an exact science; and that all things are relative. For example, it is easy to say that gravity is scientific. It is repeatable, it can be measured, and it exists throughout our known universe, yet even that is relative! Gravity on the moon is remarkably different from gravity on the earth. The studies about ulcers created and then proved opinions, or thoughts, and became established "facts"; yet, those facts were replaced by new ones a decade later! So, what is a fact?

You could postulate the following "fact": On Tuesday mornings, between 9 a.m. and 10 a.m., in New Guinea, when no one is watching, all pigs can fly. This cannot be disproved, but does that make it a fact? Can there be a false fact, and if so, who is to determine its authenticity? The definition of a fact can be argued; what is thought to be known can be altered in a minute, making room for that which is and now was known to be outdated in the next moment. What is unknown cannot be proved or disproved, and ultimately, if everything is eventually updated and proved outdated, one could conclude that all that appears to be known is really unknowable.

The more I study physics, the more
I am drawn to metaphysics.
—*ALBERT EINSTEIN, PHYSICIST*

Even the most seemingly solid aspects of sciences—or at least the interpretation of the data they present—can be flawed. Magnetic resonance imaging (MRI) shows a herniated disc which might lead your chiropractor to recommend a series of treatments based on this finding, or fact, to relieve your pain. The MRI is indisputable; it is a picture of the disc from the inside out and can be repeated. But the more empowering question is: "What does the presence of that herniated disc mean?"

It means what you or your practitioners decide it means. That is the immense power of the mind! If the interpretation of data is not something that serves you, you can decide not to give in to that system and find another. If this sounds far-fetched, look at people who were told they had six months to live, then lived for a number of years beyond that. Somewhere in their heart of hearts, they decided that the prognosis of a six-month lifespan did not serve them; they consciously chose another reality, and many times they lived that reality.

This *Theory Decides What Can Be Observed* is the only reason that all of this can make any sense—the only thing to explain the hundreds, if not thousands, of different explanations for just about anything.

So, just how important is belief? What do you believe?

In the beginning, it is believed, there was nothing. Scientists believe that the Big Bang (a massive explosion of energy) formed the stars and the planets, and eventually, humans. Some religionists believe that an all-powerful, all-knowing, yet somehow judgmental being created a world of matter made up of energy in six days, then needed a day to rest. (A six-day workweek? No thanks!) The Iroquois believe that man was cooked in an oven: with the lighter ones cooked less, the darker ones cooked more, and those in between just right. Every culture has a creation story of some kind, but which is correct? All and none of them, of course. There have been lots of things said, written, and then believed to be true, way beyond who or what created us and how. But instead of focusing on the differences and judging which stories are right and which are wrong, let us examine the underlying current of truth in all of them, and how we can use this truth to heal.

Everything around and within you is energy; that which you can see and touch is vibrating slower than that which you can hear, and that which you can hear is vibrating slower than that which you cannot perceive at all. What you perceive (or not) is only a reflection of the frequency, or the speed, at which something vibrates. According to the first law of thermodynamics, energy can neither be created nor destroyed—the amount of energy in the Universe is and always has been a constant. The only thing that changes is the form that it takes. All energy vibrates a particular frequency. Say, I'm an 8673892 and you're a 3274983, and that desk is a 420841 (the exact numbers are irrelevant; they're merely representations of arrangements of atoms forming what appears to be matter). Sound is also a frequency, say the piano playing an E is a 421384984 and a child's laughter is 8214898621; these things are not visible, yet they are within range of our five senses. The same is true with other things we take for granted, such as the smell of Grandma's pound cake and the breeze that gently sways the tree leaves. Everything vibrates at a particular frequency, whether we can acknowledge it with our five senses or not. And through it all, energy has always been the one constant.

If we can see that we are really energy vibrating at a certain frequency, it will explain how years' worth of headaches, neck, or back pain can be eliminated in much less time than previously accepted. It is easier to manipulate this energy, or the building blocks, than what you once thought of as matter to catalyze a shift in the physical. It is easier to move bits of sand than the whole beach at once. Energy is, of course, highly malleable; matter, as it has been perceived until now, is practically immovable. For that reason, mind-body healing is often quicker than physical healing modalities. The precursor to this rapid shift is transforming thought, the engine that moves energy.

We think we see a solid object, and by the laws of the physical universe, the macrocosm, that is true. And yet if we look deeply within any solid object—using an electron microscope, for example—we see another world where the laws of the physical domain no longer apply. We see energy moving in the form of atoms, electrons, protons, and so on. And if we look even farther within, we see another new world, that of quarks and leptons, the quantum layers of existence—the microcosm! This is where all the fun is. This quantum layer produces phenomena that make no sense to the macrocosm in which we usually live; yet, denying this quantum reality has led us to the current state of disharmony we now call *living*. However, to an unbiased eye, it would be more accurate to call this state, *dying*.

Our five senses trick us and hold us back from living in awareness and connection, but for good reason. All things are relative. For our very survival, we need to be able to distinguish "up" from "down," "hot" from "cold," and so on. We need to understand the **macro**cosm (the material world of the five senses) in order to access the **micro**cosm (the world of energy contained within the macrocosm). In other words, we must first learn to successfully use our five senses in order to use our other senses, such as clairvoyance (clear seeing) and clairaudience (clear hearing). We need to know "war" before we know "peace," and while the former has been the state of mind and history for millennia, it's time we look beyond that which is commonly known and accepted as the only reality. With the potential destruction of everything at the whim of almost any world leader who doesn't know or doesn't want to recognize our innate connection, this information is beyond vital. It's absolutely mandatory if we want to survive.

Everything you see and do not see is made up of energy, and all of it is affected by anything it comes in contact with, from thought to physical matter. Indeed, even the most ardent of scientists will recognize that atoms react to each other with movement and an exchange of energy and information when in the presence of other atoms. If we can accept that our building blocks are energy, atoms, and information, we can take this concept into a much bigger context to understand and improve health and illness.

We ingest a higher vibration of energy while eating an organic apple than when smoking a cigarette: one is completely natural and vibrates quickly; the other is laced with toxic chemicals and vibrates slowly. Raw foods vibrate higher than cooked foods—fruits and vegetables, more than cooked animal flesh. Organic foods vibrate even higher because they are not altered with chemicals: pesticides, by definition, carry with them the energy of death!

Of course, foods have an effect on your energy level but not as much as once thought. If you've ever said to yourself "I'm tired" more than a few times in a short period of time, you've increased the feelings of being tired—no matter what you've eaten! You can often recharge by taking a nap, but that doesn't work for everyone; some people feel no more energized than before. It is actually activity that wakes you up, not sleep. Ask anyone who works out regularly. Their energy levels will consistently be higher than that of a person who is inactive and sedentary. Even workout fiends have moments where they are tired after a long day at work, and will just want to go home and crash on the couch, but they know that all it takes is a few minutes of exercise and they'll get a second wind. After a good workout, they will be physically and mentally energized. They'll wake up the next day fully recharged, having slept better in quality and less in quantity.

Each person's energy is affected by their thoughts as well as by the thoughts of others! Your energy levels will be raised if you are near persons of good character and lowered when near those who thrive on belligerence. It is more intense when this energy is nearby than when it is farther away, but there are those who can sense things in others at quite a distance. Have you ever thought of someone and gotten a phone call from them a few minutes later? They were calling you even before they were actually calling you!

An energetic matrix links all living and nonliving things. People who see this energetic matrix often refer to it as an "aura." Others feel it on a more visceral level. Have you ever known just by a feeling in your gut that another person wasn't well—regardless of their physical proximity? Have you sensed things before they were about to happen? This is all part of the energetic matrix that is constantly being formed and re-formed with the creative power of each person's thoughts.

Have you ever stepped into a room where the air was so thick you felt like you could cut it with a knife? That tension is a result of the collective emotional states of the persons inside. Their interactions, though constantly re-created, have a tendency toward what could be called the negative. Persons in an individual and group negative mindset can drain your energy. Because they are not aware of how to channel energy from Source, they're draining each other, and perhaps even you. You can prevent being drained with conscious awareness and a mantra that calls upon the Universe for support.

NOTE: *Energy mantra: I am part of the Universe. I utilize energy from the highest Source, of which I am already a part.*

Air Supply—It Isn't Just a Band Anymore

Breathing requires the exchange of gasses in a mutually beneficial system for plants and humans. The energetic exchange is no different. Source is there for us to call upon and utilize.

Because we are energy in motion, and energy is omni-directional and never ending, you will always attract energy in alignment with your thoughts. And the laws of attraction do not differentiate between desires and fears, so think, speak, and act consciously! An example:

Late one evening, my friend and I were riding in a virtually empty subway car when a large man got on, seeming belligerent and out of touch with what most will call "reality." Okay, he was really drunk. My friend was truly terrified, so I told him to send the stranger love, because I assumed that, ultimately, that's what the stranger was missing. Within about a minute, this man completely ignored me and got right up to my friend's face starting an angry verbal assault. I was tempted to get in the way physically, but decided that to avoid an altercation I needed to send him even more love! I focused on this man intently, sending forgiveness and compassion, and reminded my friend to do the same. Eventually, he walked away.

The relevance and implications of these laws of attraction are never ending. How would you live differently knowing that every thought you have either attracts or repels the very things you want and don't want? How would you treat others, knowing that they are extensions of you?

CHAPTER 22

The New Paradigm of Healthcare:
Healing with Source

Mediocre men (persons), must, out of necessity,
have a mediocre idea of what constitutes greatness.
—*LEO TOLSTOY, AUTHOR*

We are all born with and use the ability to communicate with Guardian Angels, Spirit Guides, and alike, but within a few years are conditioned into disbelieving them. We're told that our invisible friends aren't real, and sometimes we learn to fear them. This unconscious funneling of thought invites you to live in mediocrity with the rest of the world's version of reality, with only humans and other physical beings as associates. That's too bad, because those in the spirit world, besides having access to much wisdom, are often very funny!

We replace those internal spirit–child conversations with external ones: media, gossip, worry, and our own incessant mind ramblings. How many of us can remain in silence, with or without another person, and be relaxed about it? Do you ever feel a need to talk, even if there's nothing in particular on your mind to share? Many chat on their cell phone while waiting for the bus or listen to an MP3 player while walking down a quiet street just to avoid the sounds of silence. All great musicians know that it is the silence between the sounds that makes a piece of music emotive to the listener.

You can turn off these now familiar distractions and once again access your old friends from other realms. They won't be mad at you, call you a flat-leaver, or tell you to go find some other spirit to play with. They'll welcome you like a dog does when you return from a long trip (*sans* the drool, of course) and be excited you've once again found them! There are several methods to access them. Among the most effective method is meditation.

The M Word

The only Zen you find on the tops of mountains is the Zen you bring up there.
—ROBERT M. PIRSIG, AUTHOR OF "ZEN AND THE ART OF MOTORCYCLE MAINTENANCE"

Like learning a new language, (which you are doing here), meditation is a process, and all processes require patience. As with anything new, some of you may find that you try to do it for years, with no success, while others of you will feel like you were almost born with the ability. Be assured: meditation can be done by anybody at anytime. If I can do it, you can, too. I am no different from you.

NOTE: *Prayer is the calling; meditation is the listening.*

An important thing to note here is that meditation can be a completely different process for everyone. It is not only the sit-with-your-legs-folded, silent, waiting-for-enlighten-ment on a mountaintop that we often envision. Meditation can be when you are so en-gulfed in a particular activity that nothing else seems to matter. Do you have an activity that can make you lose track of time or ignore the need to eat? These are meditations in their own way.

I figured it out long ago; it doesn't matter if you figure it out.
We all end up in the same place eventually. The rivers run
into the sea, and the sea is never filled... So I... stare out
the window. Go with the rhythm. Be in the now.
—P. BALLENTINE, AUTHOR

Anything you do that comes joyfully and without a care in the world better allows you to align with the higher forces of existence. In this state, you are more open to writing, singing, painting, making love, and being fully in the moment. When writing this book, the best information emerged when I was in a meditative state. When my Ego was at play, my thoughts lacked inspiration, if anything came out at all! In contrast, when in that connected, meditative state, you are not concerned with others' thoughts about you, your own thoughts about your past, or worries about the future. At these times, the only moment you recognize is NOW. All other moments are irrelevant because the NOW is so delicious!

This bliss is a perfectly natural state to be in. When you do more things that bring you to bliss, you become more focused, centered, and better able to accomplish things in less time. Whether this is writing the perfect sonata, drawing the greatest new car design, or making the best tofu casserole is irrelevant. At that moment, you are in bliss. At that moment, you are divinity. And when you are feeling divine, don't you think you'll be healthier than before you were feeling that way?

The Universe is filled with unconditionally loving healing energy that you can call upon on your own. While some people will want to empower themselves and take the steps in this book, others will surrender to what they feel is their higher power. Just as in a 12-step recovery program, we might admit we are powerless because we are in too deep. Neither is wrong, or bad, or even better than another. They both get results.

To call upon Source or any other nonphysical entity requires a releasing of the Ego. Watch out, though: the Ego will try to convince you not to ask for guidance. It'll call you helpless and make you feel weak for asking. In the new paradigm of healing, asking for help is a standard practice. One of the reasons I'm so effective at what I do is because I know I'm not the one doing it! I ask for help all the time. And when I can defer to Source, not only do I transmit its messages and healing energy well but you get better results. It took me a while to understand that and Source itself (not that I totally understand her in this moment), but I, like Socrates, know enough to know that I know only of my ignorance. At my "How to Communicate with Source" workshops, participants learn practical methods for calling upon Source for information, healing, and love. Until then, please trust me that Source is more than willing to lend a helping hand. And do you know what else? It has a great sense of humor! (I just heard, "flattery will get you everywhere, Dave.") See what I mean?

Okay, let's play *Jeopardy*!
You: *I'll take Unknown Truth for $2,000*
Alex: *The Answer is: According to Voltaire, he is a comic playing to an audience that is afraid to laugh.*
You: *What is God?*
Alex: *That is correct for $2,000! Nice job!*
(Audience applauds)

Humans deserve to live a life where joy and love are the norm because you and the Creator are made up of the same stuff, and Source is joy and love. Source is a Universal Consciousness; energy in vibration just like you. We vibrate slowly enough to be seen, and Source vibrates at the highest frequency that can not be seen, heard, or touched by our five senses, but she can be felt. When you meditate in silence, you invite Source into you and his presence is felt. You are then more in touch with love, or the Source/God/Goddess that already resides within you!

There is an essence of the divine in all living things.
And each person is literally a microcosm of the universe.
—*GLORIA STEINEM, EDITOR, AUTHOR*

Nature is the Best Teacher

The innate intelligence of Source's creations teach us so much, but only if we open to seeing it. We know that one of the primary causes of ill health is resistance to the flow of life (AKA Ego). We often think that something should be a certain way and get upset when it isn't—as if we know best. Nature beautifully exemplifies for us the necessary flexibility to achieve internal harmony.

When water is blocked, it builds up pressure just like we do, and the pressure must be released. As the clouds release water when they are saturated, so do humans burst at the seams when we've had enough bottling up of emotions. Water, however, doesn't demand that trees move to another neighborhood, nor does it need to move the things that are blocking it in the stream. If it comes upon a few rocks in the stream, it molds itself around the rocks and simply keeps on flowing.

Trees don't hunch over and cross their branches in frustration when they don't get enough water. They "know" that the rain will come. When the wind blows their branches to the side, barring extreme and repetitive situations, they gently spring back to their original position after the wind slows down. Plants don't kill other plants to get more sun than their neighboring plants; they too "know" that the sun's light can be shared. But humans change the weather with air conditioning and indoor heat. Some cut down trees, kill wildlife as a "sport" (how "sporting" is killing a defenseless animal with a rifle from hundreds of feet away or even a helicopter?), strip forests, and even kill other people for money, land, food, or national or religious pride. We take from others, and do so at any cost, just to have not only what we think we need now but what we fear we'll be without in the future.

God's plan for us is always bigger than our plans for us.
—*OPRAH WINFREY*

And yet if all of the world's resources, food, water, shelter, and even money were divided up equally among the inhabitants of Mother Earth, everyone would have enough! For now at least, there is enough of everything. Only our own "lack consciousness" makes us take more than we give. This, in turn, creates *haves* and *have-nots*. And as long as that remains, there will be trouble and strife. If we shared everything and gave away what we do not use, there would be more unity and peace.

As much as we have been able to develop technology and resources or grow them from the earth, there is a saturation point. Unless we're ready to boldly go where no man has gone before and start colonizing other worlds or even our own upper atmospheres, we may need to start talking about the taboo subject of population control. No one is suggesting a mandatory sterilization program; quite the opposite. What we need is dialogue and understanding. As in all things, we need to ask the "why" of everything we've yet to question.

Many people want to see their lineage continue, whether it's a last name, nationality, culture, or religion. All are illusions because death doesn't exist, and we're all the same. I am not advocating not having children; I am just pleading that we plan our families consciously. There are millions of orphans worldwide who could use your love.

GROW With the FLOW!

We can hurdle perceived obstacles if we accept that they are there, and then work around them as a river does. By going with the flow of life, we immediately reduce stress and the possibility of bursting at the seams. In fact, we'd never be that full. If we accept that there is more to life than what we think we want, how much resistance would that release?

We are made up of roughly 70–90 percent water, but we let the rest of our being dictate our lives. Water reacts at the molecular level to thoughts and energy. As shown by Dr. Masuro Emoto, author of *Messages in Water*, if water is exposed to negative energy—thoughts of war, for example—the crystals become murky. If sung to with love, water creates beautiful crystals. And we are no different. Positive thoughts of love and compassion create high vibrational energy within us, giving us internal peace, unbridled energy, and optimal health. And when we invite the highest source of love into our lives, well, what do you think will happen?

The new paradigm in healing recognizes that it is not only energy and intention but Source itself that heals; it is only us that need to allow it to happen. Most people know this intrinsically. During my Healing with Source sessions, clients experience this for themselves. And during my workshops, they learn ways of doing this work with friends, family, and the world. One of the keys to Healing with Source is the power of intention.

I know my heart is in the right place; I'm the one who put it there.
—CARRIE FISHER, ACTOR

In my experience, the intention of a "healer" is of utmost importance. If you are getting a massage from someone who just had a fight with her boyfriend, how loving is her touch going to be? If your HMO primary care physician finds it necessary to see as many people an hour as possible, how good is your care going to be? A chiropractor/acupuncturist once told me that healing is transferred from his consciousness to that of the patient *via* the acupuncture needles, that he could even assist a patient in healing by placing the needles alongside the body!

An example, though not medically related, on the power of intention: One day I theorized I could heat up a quarter while it rested on someone else's arm. I believed that by moving the energy in and around it with my hands and mind, it would happen. The first time I tried it, the person said she felt heat all over her body. Though not the desired result, I knew I was onto something. The next person did feel the heat from the quarter, and the person after that not only felt heat but a tingling all through his hand. I had no training in magic or anything like that, just a hunch and an intention.

I once demonstrated this at a lecture without even moving my hands above or anywhere near the person who had a quarter on her arm. I announced to the room that it was my intention to heat up the quarter, then began to talk about other things. Within thirty seconds, she said she felt it!

As I said above, for a practitioner intention is everything. But your intention can only be felt by Source if you can tuck away your Ego, for it is the Ego that thinks it's separate from everything and everyone. At the moment of surrender, you are your client, your client is you, you are the Source and it is you, and you are left with nothing but channeling the healing force of all that is!

> *Neither a lofty degree of intelligence nor imagination nor both together*
> *go into the making of genius. Love, love, love, that is the soul of genius.*
> —WOLFGANG AMADEUS MOZART, CLASSICAL COMPOSER

When someone who does healing work is open to utilizing Source, she is better able to facilitate healing. She can call on the highest force, or Love, and therefore know that anything is possible. At the same time, a recipient's ability to heal directly correlates with their willingness to receive healing energy. It's important that the healing practitioner advise the recipient of all possibilities in a healing session, so that they are fully informed and open to all or nothing happening. Sometimes, people have what might be called a miraculous experience. Other times, it will seem like nothing at all is happening. But we must trust that something is shifting, and given time and patience, all will become clear.

Healing can be blocked if the recipient so wishes, perhaps out of an unconscious fear of being proved wrong. Some traditional practitioners will not be too excited about reading this text. They may not believe in mind-body medicine, and that's fine. They will continue to attract those persons who need their particular healing assistance, and everyone will be all the better for it. "For everything (everyone) there is a purpose." They may recommend drugs for symptom X, and the side effects we'll call Y are worse than those of symptom X that you were trying to help. Then you will take another drug to help with Y, and that drug, too, will have side effects that we'll call Z. You will now have X, Y, and Z!

Side effects, by the way, while they certainly can come from any physical properties in the medication, can also be an end result of the negative energy that any given drug may already have within it or that which is created by the person taking the medication, especially if they are ingesting it in a state of anger. "I wish I didn't need this damn medication," or perhaps it reminds them of the illness that they'd prefer to forget. Always ingest with gratitude. Would you rather the medication not be available? It is a vicious cycle when the focus is on symptoms alone. Ultimately, healing happens from within, but it's perfectly okay to get a little help on the way.

> *I wake up in the morning, and I consciously create my day the way*
> *I want it to happen. When I create my day, out of nowhere, little things*
> *happen that are so unexplainable, I know that they are the process or the*
> *result of my creation. And the more I do that, the more I build a neural net,*
> *in my brain, I accept that that's possible.*
> —JOSEPH DISPENZA, D.C., FROM "WHAT THE BLEEP DO WE KNOW?"

Sometimes we don't erase, we rewrite. The past is merely a memory that can be rewritten to a better outcome. With the help of a good practitioner, you can go back in time in your mind and actually change the past. Listen to any two people talking about an earlier event and you'll hear two different realities around it. Add in a third person, and you've got three versions. So, who's got the right one? They're all right! You can pick one of them and let it sink into your cells. Some time after that, it becomes your reality, too, and the stream of consciousness that energizes your life will also be changed. Say you were really hurt by someone a long time ago. In your mind, you can go back in time and change what happened. You can dump them before they dump you! You can quit before being fired. You can choose forgiveness instead of choosing revenge.

It is irrelevant to the body if this new version is real or not; your body responds as if it's true. This is the power of the mind-body connection! Just like crying at the sad movie, within seconds your body will react to whatever thoughts you may have. Change one scenario for the better in your mind on your own, now feel how your body reacts. Now take it into a larger perspective and consciously create a memory you previously only wished for, and see what happens. You can create your day as well as create your past! How do you think that'll affect your future?!

He is the best physician who is the most ingenious inspirer of hope.
—*SAMUEL TAYLOR COLERIDGE, POET*

My grandmother used to swear by Dr. Klein; no matter what you had, you felt better when you left his office. Dr. Klein took time to discuss with his patients all they needed to know to understand about their illness. His gift was compassion and inspiring hope. In my experience, all practitioners truly wish that their clients will get better, but it is their scope of practice that has imposed the limits. When practiced without attachment to an end result, Healing with Source is limited only by the degree to which we believe in its efficacy. It's that simple.

CHAPTER 23

Practical Applications of Healing with Source

By now it should be clear that nothing can be reversed without fully understanding and transforming the causative energy. So let us review what we've already learned, and then expand into practical healing applications.

The steps for healing acute pain and illness are similar to the steps for prevention, which much of the preceding text has focused on. There's an added sense of urgency, perhaps, but the concepts are the same. It's never too late to open your heart and forgive. If you've been carrying around back pain for example, you can never truly heal (at the core and with permanence) by focusing on the symptom. As you think about and even address the back pain, you are giving more energy to back pain, thus reinforcing or even exacerbating what you do not want.

However, what's making itself known is much more than the pain itself. It is forcing you to take a time out and get a fresh, more spiritual and holistic understanding of what's going on in your life. In this case, is the pain really a burden? No, of course not, it's an opportunity for healing being shown to you through a message that's hard to miss! While you may go into, "I don't want this pain," or even an "I shouldn't have this pain," I can tell you from first-hand experience and from that of my clients, that is exactly the opposite of healing at the Source.

Let's say the Tools to Raise Awareness from Chapter 3 have helped you determine that the chronic pain in your lower back is from repressed anger toward your father. You have been carrying around this burden as a result of your perception that he was not there for you when you were younger. Once the awareness of the cause has formed in your mind's eye, let the reversal of that cause, not the back pain or even the elimination of the back pain, be your focus. Now use the Five Steps to Health as described in Chapter 4.

Be aware of the underlying cause. Work with accepting that this perception of Dad's absence has manifested in the lower-back pain, and that you caused/created this perception and manifestation, even unconsciously. Take responsibility. See it as an opportunity, not a burden. See this moment as a gift, and express gratitude for the message. And then work diligently at forgiving him.

Notice that none of the Five Steps say to focus on healing the back pain; yet, by doing this work, your back pain will heal at the causative level. It won't come back days, months, or years later, as happens when using just about all medications, or even many surgeries.

So how does one Heal with Source? Once you truly get that Source can be called upon for healing, you have to create "safe space" for your friend or client, which happens when you release your Ego. Set intention, trust your intention will happen, and trust that the process and the end results may or may not look anything like you expect. Source likes to keep us on our toes, and as frustrating as that can be to our minds, our soul knows the bigger picture. Tap into the soul, which is having fun no matter what your mind and body are doing, and open up to the possibility that Source knows more than we do. Let it do its thing!

Create safe space for healing. That includes allowing yourself to have absolutely no judgments about the process, the recipient, or even yourself. Know that each person is on their path, to the point where all judgments are dropped. Knowing everyone is where they're supposed to be will make it easier to forgive others' transgressions. It's not up to you to fix them, but it is up to you to love them.

You can self-heal with this, of course, but everything is better when shared. We're going to focus on both sharing and receiving Source's healing energy so that you can heal and also become an effective energy healing practitioner. What you send out is always returned, so by working with others, you're also working on yourself! This book is a powerful tool to help.

I was told by Source that a famous artist in New York City would channel a symbol of God's love for others to heal at the same energetic frequency that I currently use. When I spoke with her she said, "Oh, so you're the one who I've been doing this for!" This symbol is extremely powerful. She said it was difficult to draw because of the power it was transmitting and took her much longer than anything else she'd done that was similar. This symbol is found on page 173, and anyone can use it, anywhere, any time. Its efficiency is relative to:

- the awareness and spiritual development of the giver and to some degree, the receiver;
- the willingness of the giver to truly be in service; and
- the willingness and receptivity of the receiver to the healing

You can even self-heal with this symbol. In this case, your openness to see things in a new light is key. And again, this self-healing process is strengthened by your working with the concepts within these pages.

When you know what your core issue is and have done the Five Steps, gently cut out the Healing with Source symbol on page 173 and place it on the affected area. Let yourself open to God's love. In fact, the message the artist heard while drawing it was, "God's Love is All." Think about your core issue and let yourself feel. Involve more than one sense—whatever it takes to feel something viscerally—so include sound to your process. While the symbol is on the affected area, pretend you're a kid again. Without caring about rhyme or meter or even relative pitch, let yourself make up a song.

Let's say the problem is lower-back pain arising from feeling unsupported by your father, as mentioned above. Make up a song about how caring your father was. Chant or sing how he tried his best, and only did what he thought was good for you. Remember that no matter how unloving his actions may have been, somewhere deep within him there is love for you. Let yourself feel that love, and send forgiveness energy to him. Sing to his inner child, which is likely be in a lot of pain. He needn't be in the room, city, or even alive for you to do this. The "God's Love is All" symbol will amplify this message to whoever it needs to go to. Sound odd? At one time, people believed the earth was flat, too. At another time, people used bloodletting for many illnesses. And many years ago, it was thought to be impossible to communicate with people on other continents, in other countries, or even nearby towns. And now we carry that technology in our pockets.

Do this healing process twice a day for 10 minutes each, once in the morning and once at night. You can always do more if you feel called to do so. Try to set up consistent start times and stick to it as best as possible. If you can't self-heal at that time one day, don't beat yourself up. Just do your best.

When working with another person, do it for 30 minutes at a time as often as possible each week. Place the symbol on their affected area, and place your hands over the symbol. Both of you should focus on healing the issue, not the ailment. Always focus on the underlying cause because if you focus on the ailment—which is what you've already done with no permanent success—you're giving energy to the symptom. And what you focus on expands.

Depending on the depth of the cause, and the willingness to release it, you may only need to do this a few times. If there is resistance, it can take a lot longer. However long it takes, just do it. What have you got to lose? Twenty or 30 minutes a day? And if you think about it, can anything bad ever happen when sending forgiveness energy to another person? Of course not. BUT...

Yes, the proverbial but...

Your Ego will make the healing process more and more difficult. It doesn't want you to heal. So you'll have to love your way through the pitfalls and roadblocks it'll set up for you. Don't be dismayed or let it win! Your health depends on it. Treat the process as if it means everything to you. Address it like you would any worthwhile goal—know that this process works.

While this may seem far-fetched, notice that what you have been doing hasn't worked. Be open to something new. Ask yourself, "From whom did I learn my version of reality?" Perhaps you'll list parents, schoolteachers, mass media, or society. To quote author Gregg Braden, "Well, what if they're wrong?"

It's not our intention to label anything right or wrong—more, it's to focus on effective healing. I don't believe anything is intrinsically wrong, especially if it leads you to a deeper understanding. In that case, everything labeled as wrong is really a first-hand teaching device that expands our version of reality.

I say *our version of reality* because as we said earlier, for any event there are numerous interpretations. Note that on this earth right now, there are more than 6 billion versions of reality. And every one of your 3 trillion cells has a memory. That means that at any given second there are at least 18,000,000,000,000,000,000,000 versions of reality. Don't you think some of those will be more empowering than others? Lucky us, we get to choose. And even more fortunate, we have teachers—some obvious, some not—along the way.

Sometimes it's helpful to have a visual image of forgiveness and the absence of anger. Check out the Dalai Lama! Stare into the eyes of a baby, a puppy, or a statue of Buddha. Forgiveness is the correction of perception. You've been living a version of reality that has been blaming others, perhaps even being angry at them, too, and this critical way of behaving has come back to bite you in the butt, or in the back, or wherever you're experiencing pain. I invite you to look at it as a love bite, a kick in the pants that wakes you up to a happier life and not this overbearing burden that others have placed upon you. There is no other way to truly heal.

Remember that things in the conscious mind only become habit through repetition. This is no different. When you do enough forgiveness work and can finally have a conversation with your parents while looking at them the way you wanted to be seen when you were younger, then you know you're onto something. Even if they're no longer in the physical body, you can do the same with a picture, or even just a mental image. Always note that what you send out is given back to you. As you love unconditionally, others will begin to do the same back to you. And it could be argued that all pain and illness come from not being loved unconditionally. So if that's at the root of everything, why would you want to pick a few berries off the branches when working at the root is so much more effective? Sure, it's tough, but who said it would be easy? It's tough being here in the 3D world, but with awareness of what's really going on, that perception of difficulty can be minimized. You really can live better than you ever have by sending out that which you always wanted, unconditional love.

Let's take another example. You've discovered that your colon, lungs, or skin ailments have been caused by the repression of grief. Remember the earlier chapters that said grief can be our friend? Every time we cry, whether from laughing or sadness, we are shedding one of our many layers of grief. And most of you wouldn't believe the amount of grief in your bodies if it were shown to you in a tangible form. It's pervasive! You know that every time you cry, you feel better afterward—is that not a part of healing in itself?

Many of us have an underlying sense of grief in our day-to-day existence. Some of us let it out and others don't, either because you don't feel safe to or because you're afraid that once you do so, the feelings of grief will never end. I assure you that the latter isn't true. In fact, by releasing the feelings of grief when possible, you're decreasing the amount in the body and, of course, the ever-present feeling of sadness begins to fade. The average intense emotion only lasts three minutes. Just three minutes can release underlying causative energies if you really let it rip!

Now, how many of you are thinking, "What? He wants me to just start crying? *That's* gonna shed my illness?" Well, as effective as crying can be, we know that it's not gonna happen for many of you just by saying, "Okay, I think I'll start crying now"

And this is where the true beauty of the Source can be seen and felt.

Whatever is needed, Source will help you with if you let it. I've worked with people who have had decades of grief stored in their bodies so intensely that their energy level is low (of course, it gets tiring holding everything in for so long). In the West, it's called chronic fatigue syndrome—just another label that disables. Others get through what is called depression in a similar way. They didn't shed a tear, but their symptoms vanished within a few months' time. We invited Source to release it for us.

While that may seem ridiculous, experience shows me it's real. Think of Source as a good friend. Wouldn't a good friend remove your grief if he or she knew how? The only condition required is that you surrender your fear of releasing it, open up to the gifts of grace, and be willing to feel uncomfortable for a bit. The latter would make sense; if you've been storing up years of sadness, it makes sense that when it comes out it'll be uncomfortable, and yet it doesn't have to be. *Willingness is the cosmic grease of healing, and commitment is the motor.* When you are willing to feel whatever needs to be felt, more space is created for quick release. When you are committed to healing, the Universe supports you. How do you show commitment? By acting from love not fear, showing compassion not apathy, and by living The Five Steps!

So you can see there are many variables, and as much as your mind wants instructions like *Step 1, followed by Step 2, and for how long each is to be applied,* that is not the way true healing happens. Rooted in the concept of holism is that everyone is different. And as frustrating as your mind might find that, it is a whole lot more frustrating following rules and regimens espoused elsewhere that you're told will work but really don't.

So what about if you've got a tumor? Western medicine will likely remove it—a good thing. But is that a healing thing? No. In most cases, the tumor comes back—sometimes in another area. It'll seem unrelated, but nothing is unrelated; everything is connected. For those who appear healed with no reoccurrences, I guarantee you they've gotten the message of this book, perhaps without having read it. They've been awakened by a brush with fear, perhaps their own mortality stared them in the face, and now they've shifted their life to one of more love, forgiveness, and understanding of how precious every breath is. My intention is for you to get this message **before** you have to face those frightening conditions.

Few of the pains or illnesses that I work with are new. In fact, as you commit to healing yourself, old pains will resurface. They will seem to come out of nowhere, but that is the farthest from the truth. More opportunities have arisen, and it's up to you to take them on. There may be times where things are so uncomfortable that you'll want out. "Okay, God, I was just kidding. This hurts too much; I want to go back to living in ignorance. At least I was happy then." Sure, ignorance is bliss, but it's short lived and now that you know otherwise, you can't go back. You can try, but you can't. Because you'll see that ignorance is not blissful. It's actually a whole lot more painful than where awareness leads. At the point of frustration, reach out to someone who's been through it already, a practitioner you trust. Your true freedom exists just on the other side of this discomfort. Like a runner who hits the wall, she knows that just beyond that wall is the equivalent of turbo power! So she'll let her muscles scream in agony, her mind racing toward the finish line, and in an instant, though most likely a painful instant, the perception of a wall will be gone.

Life is not peaches and cream. There are thousands of books that say it can be, but all the authors are just as human and just as flawed and just as in the process of healing as you and me. Life may be partly peaches and cream, but it is also pain and illness, death and destruction, and loving, divine purpose. The more we hang onto ideals that say that life should be pain-free, the more pain we experience. The more we resist what is obviously so, the more resistance takes refuge in our bodies. The more resistance that is in our bodies, the more energy stagnation exists. This results in what you've been calling pain or illness, and hopefully by now can call an opportunity for growth and expansion.

While we heal the causative layers, opening to more vitality, we're also likely to feel that things will be better on the other side. *Better* is a judgment, and as long as you think over there is better than what's happening right now over here, there is less chance of getting there, enjoying the ride, and enjoying life when you are finally there. Why? Because there is no *there* to get to. And focusing on that nonexistent place takes you away from what's happening now. And now is all there is.

So what's the purpose of doing all this work? While working toward a better life, we're usually stuck in old patterns that say that joy is elsewhere. In reality, you'll be opening to more challenges! These challenges can come in the form of physical or emotional obstacles (You didn't want to hear that did you?), and it's all designed so that you grow spiritually. That is the only purpose of life, and when that spiritual growth is seen as a challenge and not a burden, there is joy! If you perceive what's happening correctly, very little will be sad, very little will bring up anger, and very little will be seen as imperfect. You may get frustrated, but that's your Ego speaking not your soul. Your soul is your connection to divinity, and God hasn't made a mistake in a very long time. When we can feel the truth of that, the perfection in everything makes itself clear.

Remember what we said in the beginning: "We most often think that health is a stationary state of being—it is not. It, like life, is a process. It is not a destination, but more a given end result from living consciously—in awareness of how things work, what is missing, and where and how to fill in those blanks." While this may frustrate you, take a look at all the pie-in-the-sky books you've read and workshops you've attended, and note that you're still looking for answers. This is a very difficult concept to accept, but acceptance will alter your entire sense of being. Your life's work may be seen as a waste of time, but it's not a waste because it brought you to this place where true healing can begin.

So, read this book again and start implementing the understandings presented. As you live with greater perception, you'll see things very differently from the way you used to do. What you were taught is that you had no power; just the opposite is true. You were taught that you are a victim of circumstance; also untrue. Within you already are truth-recognizing atoms that scream *yes!* when you read something that awakens you. If you've been reading this and nodding your head in understanding and approval, you know what I mean. If you've been shaking your head *no*, you've got more work to do. And that's okay.

I am undefeated in this game called life. A perfect record: 1–0.

As we said earlier, if you were presented the trophy before the game began, the game is over. And *in* the game of life is where all the fun occurs. It's also where all the challenges exist. Let this book challenge you. Let life challenge you. You can't find solid ground in a world made of energy where solid ground doesn't even exist, so you might as well stop searching for it. You can't know the future, so why pretend you can control it? And you can't know what will bring you joy until you've realized exactly what doesn't.

What does the support of Source look like? As you commit to deeper growth and understanding Source commits with you. I've signed up for workshops way out of my price range, and both times, because I trusted that's where I needed to be, the money showed up. And with relative ease. But the Universe conspires to work with you in ways way beyond money. Money is just energy—a way of expressing appreciation for goods and services; it can never make you happy. Commit to being happy and following your bliss—not your Ego's bliss, but that of the soul—and money finds you. In fact, whatever you need finds you! Commit to being healthy and watch as the concepts in this book come alive or practitioners make themselves known. If you don't think you have time, I dare you to add up all the hours you watch television a week, then multiply that number times 52. Now with that number of hours per year you've spent watching life instead of experiencing life blaring in front of you, ask yourself the same question.

Does this mean that it can take that many hours to heal? You betchya! Does it have to? No. It can occur overnight in some cases; it all depends on how openly you embrace what all of life is showing you. What else do you have to do? What is more important than your health and your happiness? You've been searching all along, and you're still un-healthy and not always happy. And if you think you're happy, it may be your Ego tricking you. Or you have a low expectation from life and yourself that's letting you believe that true happiness isn't possible. Readers of this book don't settle. That's for others. Consider yourself a spiritual warrior if you've gotten this far; now go deeper into your own self with these freshened perspectives. Then go out into the world and be the change you always wanted to be.

Healing with Source in a Group Format

Obviously, there are many factors involved in true healing. One that is too often over-looked is receiving support from others. This is very sad, because it's one of the most important. In fact, I'd say that support and consistency are the most important if you truly want to heal and grow.

I currently run weekly in-person Power Groups where attendees come together to practice what's in this book based on what comes to me and others in the moment, as needed. Because of the large number of people at these groups and at workshops relative to the allocated time, some participants don't get personal attention; yet, they too, grow and heal! How can this be?

What you send out is what is sent back, and I have instructed everyone in the group to be as attentive and supportive as possible. It sounds odd but if you've made it this far, you should be expecting more oddities. But I have seen this growth with my own eyes, and attendees have experienced it; we are all connected. What you do for others you are also doing for you.

Conversely, some people don't grow. And almost always that is because they're overly concerned with themselves. A powerful lesson on our interconnectedness.

Often a group format makes it easier to face our deepest issues. For most people, the two most difficult things are to ask for help and to say no. By creating safe space, people can practice these things and then take them out into the world. It makes it real easy to see what you have to work on, too. Whatever bothers you about another is something that needs work in you. And how wonderful is it to have people to push your buttons when your parents aren't around to do it for you? Annoying? Yes! Frustrating? Yes! Healing? Well, if you take on the challenges, absolutely!

By working in larger groups, I can facilitate this work to wider audiences, and we can all begin to shift at the causative levels of existence. As you open, you will see that others' experiences often mirror your own. We all want the same things, but few people know how to get them. When guided by an open vessel, magic can happen. Another thing I recommend to all participants is to write about their experience. Not only does this documentation reinforce what they're learning, it's something to look back on if they should ever fall back into old ways. Documenting the process helps to remind you that you can do this work and you can see benefits from it. Let yourself be supported by others in all your endeavors, be they healing, growth, or even manifesting a soul mate.

How do you attract those people? You guessed it! By being one of those people! As you support others, they and others will support you. They needn't be master healers or teachers to support you, just as you needn't be a master to support them. Just be there, hold space, and embody unconditional love as best you can. You have nothing to lose, well, except your ego and everything it brings, and everything wonderful to gain.

All journeys to find the self end in realizing there is no self.

www.davemarkowitz.com

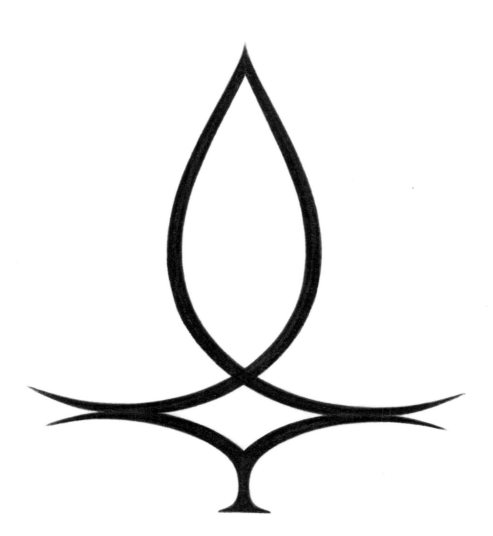

FINDHORN PRESS

Life Changing Books

For a complete catalogue,
please contact:

Findhorn Press Ltd
117-121 High Street,
Forres IV36 1AB,
Scotland, UK

t +44 (0)1309 690582
f +44 (0)131 777 2711
e info@findhornpress.com

or consult our catalogue online
(with secure order facility) on
www.findhornpress.com

For information on the Findhorn Foundation:
www.findhorn.org